Managing
Arthritis Pain

Controlling your pain successfully

Dr Jo Clough, Medical Editor

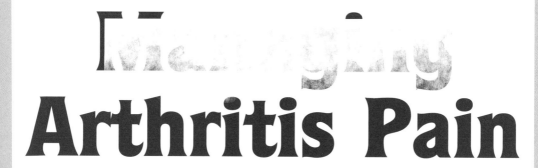

With a Foreword by
Neil Betteridge,
Chief Executive, Arthritis Care

CLASS PUBLISHING • LONDON

Feedback is welcomed from the users of this book. Please contact the publisher.

**Class Publishing (London) Ltd, Barb House, Barb Mews, London W6 7PA
Telephone: 020 7371 2119; Fax: 020 7371 2878 [International +4420]
Email: post@class.co.uk**

Notice The information presented in this book is accurate and current to the best of the author and medical editor's knowledge. They and the publisher, however, make no guarantee as to, and assume no responsibility for, the correctness, sufficiency or completeness of such information or recommendation. The reader is advised to consult a doctor regarding all aspects of individual health care.

A CIP catalogue record for this book is available from the British Library

ISBN 10: 1 85959 122 1
ISBN 13: 978 1 85959 122 3

Edited by Gillian Clarke
Indexed by Michèle Clarke
Typeset by Martin Bristow
Printed and bound in Singapore by Tien Wah Press

Original title: *The Arthritis Foundation's Guide to Pain Management*
Copyright © 2003 by the Arthritis Foundation, Atlanta, Georgia

UK edition published under arrangement with
THE ARTHRITIS FOUNDATION, Atlanta, Georgia, USA

ABOUT THE MEDICAL EDITOR

Jo Clough is a paediatric physician who specializes in asthma and allergic diseases. Until recently a senior lecturer at the University of Southampton, she is a Fellow of the Royal College of Paediatrics & Child Health, and a Member of the Royal College of Physicians. She received her DM from the University of Southampton.

Dr Clough originally trained as an anaesthetist and is a Fellow of the Royal College of Anaesthetists. She now works as a Medical Adviser and is the author of *Allergies at your fingertips* (Class Publishing).

Contents

Contents *continued*

FOREWORD

When I was a child growing up with arthritis in the 1960s, I did not have the faintest idea that you could actually do something about pain. I thought that, if tablets didn't do what it said on the label and kill the pain, you just had to put up with it.

For make no mistake, although forms of arthritis vary greatly, the one constant is pain. Pain which, if left unchallenged, can take a person of any age from independence to dependence and from a positive outlook on life to misery.

If only I had known then what I know now – that, with a careful approach to trying out new coping strategies, you really can control much of the pain and not allow it to control you.

This book has drawn together the most up-to-date knowledge available on tips and techniques to help you stay on top of the pain of arthritis. What's more, by taking contributions from Arthritis Care and others experienced in this area, the contents come to you via the real experts – those who live with arthritis and understand its impact.

Not everything will help every individual: certain horses prefer different courses. But there is something here to empower everyone with chronic or intermittent pain.

So I recommend that you read, consider and take control – it's good for you.

Neil Betteridge
Chief Executive
Arthritis Care

PREFACE

Chronic pain is a thief; it can steal your life away. This doesn't happen overnight – when your pain first arrives you have no idea that it has come to stay. But one day you find that it has taken up residence, and realize that, like a cuckoo in a nest, it has elbowed out of your life so many of the things that gave you pleasure. Both the big things – a sport, a relationship, maybe even your job – and those little things that feel big – like getting down on your hands and knees to play with a favourite child – have been affected.

Chronic pain can affect just about every aspect of your life. It may disrupt your sleep, sap your energy and take away your sparkle. The pain medications you take may give you unpleasant side effects. You may even have difficulty carrying out everyday tasks that others take for granted. Your world can become a less joyful place.

But it doesn't have to be like this!

If you can learn more about your pain – where it comes from, why and how it has become long-standing, what can make it worse, new ways of controlling it – you have made the first steps towards learning how to manage your pain so that you can live the life you want to lead.

This book can help you. It not only explains the whys and wherefores of chronic pain, it also offers a wide and comprehensive variety of strategies you can employ to help you tackle your pain. Whilst conventional medical treatments are covered in depth, this book also discusses helpful complementary therapies and self-management approaches.

Although it is written for people coping with the pain of arthritis – this condition affects over 9 million people of all ages in the UK – most of the information and advice in this book is also directly relevant to people with chronic pain caused by other conditions. It is written in a very straightforward and accessible way which will allow you to choose the approaches that are most appropriate for you and your type of pain. This is important, as every person is unique, and you yourself can become the real expert on how to manage your own condition. This book will show you how.

Dr Jo Clough

Introduction

Pain (pān) *n.* a strongly unpleasant sensation such as is caused by illness or injury

Concise Oxford Dictionary

Pain, as the dictionary defines it, seems like a simple matter. You feel hurt or uncomfortable when you have had an injury or illness. When you are experiencing pain, however, trying to describe how it feels, pinpoint its cause or find a helpful treatment are anything but easy.

Pain is one of the most common health complaints among people today. There are many different types of pain: a dull ache, a sharp stab, a recurring throb, a sudden sting, a constant burning, and many more. Pain may be caused by any number of ailments, including disease, injuries, stress and others. But a few facts are applicable when discussing any type of pain or any of pain's causes. Here are the important points to remember as you begin reading this book:

• Pain is real.

• Pain has a cause.

• Pain can impair your ability to perform your everyday activities.

• Pain is treatable.

• Pain can, in most cases, be managed.

There are many different ways to treat your pain, including new methods developed by recent medical research. However, treating pain can be a complicated process for doctors and patients. Some people may struggle to find the most effective treatment for their type of pain, particularly if they have *chronic* (long-lasting) pain. Others may find relief from their pain but suffer from unpleasant or life-disrupting side effects from pain-fighting or *analgesic* medications. In addition to drugs and other medical devices to treat pain, there are many lifestyle changes – a practice known as *self-management* – that people may make to help relieve and prevent pain. These changes may include exercise, getting proper rest, controlling stress or cutting down on drinking alcohol or smoking.

Because there are so many different causes and types of pain, and so many methods to alleviate pain, some doctors actually specialize in treating pain itself. These professionals practise in a field known as *pain medicine.* Yet you are most likely to receive attention and treatment for your pain from your GP. If you have a serious chronic illness, such as arthritis or fibromyalgia, you might receive pain treatment from the specialist (such as a *rheumatologist,* a doctor with specialized training in treating arthritis-related diseases) who treats you for that illness.

As we noted earlier, there are many health problems that can cause intense pain. The pain may be *acute* (serious, but lasting for a short time) or chronic. This book will focus mainly on causes of chronic pain and treatments for that pain, including drugs, surgery, complementary therapies, supplements and things you can do on your own, such as exercise or stress-relief techniques.

Why is chronic pain uniquely challenging? Acute pain, such as that caused by a broken bone, an ear infection or a kidney stone, can be excruciating. Yet acute pain can often be managed easily with medications, ice application, elevation and rest. Once the injury or health problem that caused the acute pain has healed, the pain is usually gone. But chronic pain, such as that caused by arthritis, is a daily occurrence. The pain may subside at times, and get suddenly worse at other times (an experience known as a *flare*), but it is always present in the person's life.

The most important first step in treating your pain is making an appointment with your doctor. Remember: pain is not something you 'just have to live with'. Your pain has a cause – something that may be a serious health problem that needs to be addressed and treated with medications and, possibly, surgery – and should be diagnosed by a doctor. Don't try to treat serious pain on your own.

In some cases, *over-the-counter* medicines (bought without a prescription) can be used to treat your mild pain. But for most people with chronic pain, or even a severe flare of pain that is usually manageable, the best option is to see a doctor. You and your doctor will create a *pain-management plan*. With this plan, you and your doctor can start treating your pain now and keep it from getting worse.

What happens if you just 'live with the pain'? Pain that continues without proper treatment affects your whole body. Your muscles might weaken, your immune system (your body's way of healing itself) can suffer, or you can become depressed. It's important that you treat your pain, and your doctor can help you.

Your doctor might not just prescribe medicine but can also suggest treatments such as heat or cold therapy, exercises, a brace or splint, and others. We will discuss all of these treatments and many more in this book. You should use this information to add to the discussions you have with your doctor – but never as a replacement for a doctor's advice and treatment.

Whether you have arthritis, fibromyalgia, bursitis or another form of recurring or chronic pain, your doctor can prescribe treatments for your pain. He or she may also prescribe treatments for the disease that is causing your pain. In other words, some drugs modify the processes in the body that may be causing your pain. By treating the disease, your symptoms, including the pain, can be alleviated.

Your doctor can provide powerful tools to fight your pain and the problems that cause it. Yet there is much that you can do on your own to control and, in some cases, prevent your pain. The person with a chronic illness must learn ways to self-manage their ongoing pain through a combination of medications and lifestyle changes. Whilst it is not necessary for you to just live with the pain or 'grin and bear it', it is necessary for you to live your life and avoid the negative consequences of chronic pain. It's that mental challenge – keeping your spirits up, avoiding negativity and focusing on something other than your pain – that can be the most difficult to meet.

This book outlines a number of strategies to relieve pain. Some strategies are medical and others involve alternative approaches to drugs and other medical methods. Something as simple as a daily stretching routine or applying a bag of ice cubes or frozen peas can help alleviate some pain. This book also contains a chapter on strategies to reduce stress (which can worsen pain) and use your mind's power to help fight pain.

Managing Arthritis Pain will offer you a great deal of information about pain and the latest ways to keep pain under control. By working with your doctor and exploring some of the strategies in this book, you should find the methods that help you. The aim of this book is to help guide you to effective methods of beating your pain, so that you can live the full, active life you deserve.

Don't let pain win this battle! We can help you take control of your pain and start living well once more.

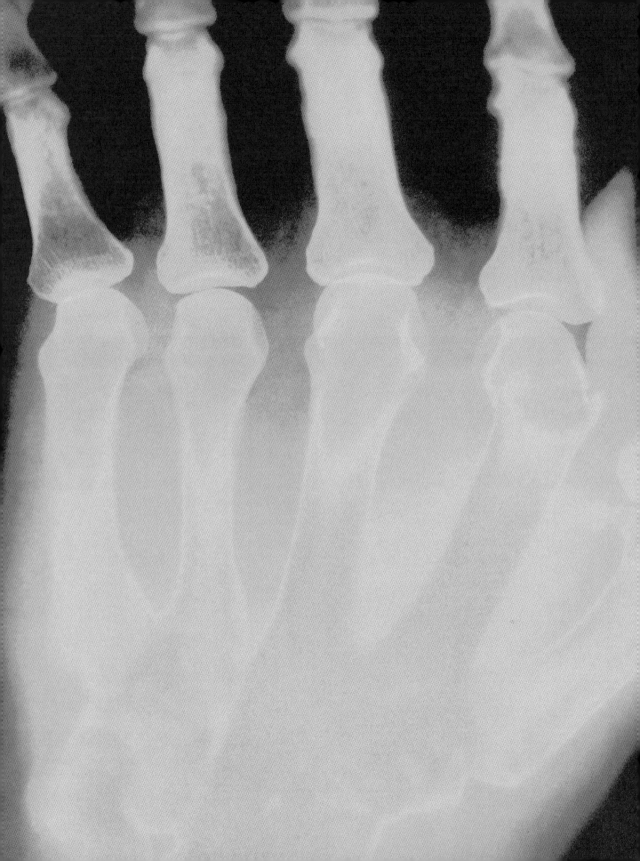

What Is Pain?

1

CHAPTER 1: WHAT IS PAIN?

Pain is not just a problem in itself. Pain is a *symptom*. Pain is the body's warning system. It's a signal from your body that something is wrong – just like a security alarm that buzzes when something goes awry. For example, if you step on a drawing pin, it is important to stop walking and remove it from your foot before it does any more damage. Pain is the body's signal that you need to take action. You can treat the pain itself but it's also important to know what may be causing the pain.

Whilst pain that lasts only a short time may be treated and then mostly forgotten, chronic or long-lasting pain – like the pain associated with arthritis, fibromyalgia, chronic back problems and similar conditions – is an alarm that keeps ringing and ringing. You feel that the pain is always there, subsiding at times and suddenly worsening at others. Pain is not only a nuisance; it may also be a clear message from your body that something is wrong. The problem causing your pain should be addressed or the pain may worsen. If you ignore the pain, the cause of the pain may progress.

If you are in pain, you are not alone. Millions of people experience some kind of pain on a regular basis, and many of them experience chronic or long-lasting pain. This type of pain, which includes the pain of arthritis, has a tremendous impact on the lives of those who have it.

The effects of pain go beyond the person experiencing it – both physically and emotionally. It also affects those close to the person and has a significant impact in terms of lost income and lost productivity because of time taken from work.

In order to help you, your doctor needs to know as much as possible about you and your condition. Some aspects are fairly easy to explain but describing your pain can be difficult. So communicating your pain to your doctor, understanding it yourself and finding the right treatments to control the pain are key.

Everyone experiences pain differently. For one person, a headache might be an annoying interruption to the workday, while another person might spend hours in bed with a cold facecloth on her forehead. Why? The intensity and nature of the first person's headache might be quite different from the headache experienced by the second person.

In addition, each person's unique psychological and physical composition – as well as gender, age and even cultural background, according to some researchers – may have an effect on how he or she perceives pain. This variance makes it more difficult for healthcare professionals to assess your pain and pinpoint the correct treatments.

There are many reasons for pain, and different categories and types of pain. In this chapter, we learn more about how pain happens, why it occurs and what physical problems may lead to serious pain.

To begin to understand why you feel pain, you must first understand an elaborate network in your body: the *nervous system*. The nervous system, masterminded by its boss, the brain, runs most of the processes in your body. Without it, you would be just a lump of flesh! The nervous system brings you to life and action. It governs every movement in your body, including those you are aware of (picking up a leaf and feeling its surface) and those you rarely notice (your heartbeat or your breathing).

The nervous system is made up of the *central nervous system*, which comprises the brain and the spinal cord, and the *peripheral nervous system*.

The peripheral nervous system is made up of two different systems: the *somatic system*, which supplies the skin and the body's musculoskeletal system; and the *autonomic nervous system*, which supplies the muscles of our internal organs.

- The somatic system allows the voluntary control of the bones, joints and skeletal muscles, all the sensations felt by them and the different sensations felt by the skin.

- The autonomic nervous system is responsible for controlling the involuntary body functions such as the beating of the heart, breathing, sweating, blood pressure and digestion of food.

These two systems function together, with nerves from the periphery entering and becoming part of the central nervous system, and vice versa.

HOW PAIN HAPPENS

Pain, as we said earlier, is almost like a fire alarm ringing in your body. When you feel pain, what you are really experiencing is an elaborate communication and response effort between the nerves, the spinal cord and the brain.

In your body, there is an elaborate network of millions of nerve cells around your body. Nerves are located all over your skin, in your bones, joints and muscles, and around internal organs, such as your stomach or liver. The individual nerve cells wind together into nerves, and these nerves communicate with other parts of the nervous system.

The specialized endings of the sensory (feeling) nerve fibres are called *receptors*; they change physical and chemical signals into messages. Different sensory nerves have different functions – some sense light touch and vibration, others cold, pressure and heat. Some nerve endings, the *nociceptors*, sense the presence of tissue damage, often a symptom of arthritis, probably via the production of certain chemicals such as prostaglandins and substance P and produce the sensation of pain.

Nociceptors are tiny: it takes more than 1,000 nociceptors to cover an area of your skin the size of a postage stamp. There are more nociceptors in some parts of your body than others, which is why some areas of your body are more sensitive than others. Your skin and exposed membranes such as your eyes have more nerve endings. Body parts such as muscles and bones, protected beneath your skin, have fewer nociceptors, and the coverings of your internal organs have even fewer. Chronic pain felt in your bones, joints and muscles can be strong even though there are fewer nerve endings there than in highly sensitive areas such as the tips of your fingers.

How Nerves Feel Pain

Let's take the example of touching a very hot stove with your finger.

First, the damaged tissue releases a number of different chemicals, including histamine and substance P. These stimulate the *nociceptors* (pain receptors) in the skin. Pain signals are sent from these receptors via sensory (feeling) nerves to the spinal cord. Here, the signals are processed by an area of the spinal cord called the *dorsal horn*, and an automatic reflex to pull your hand away from the heat is generated and sent down the motor nerves to the arm. This reflex does not involve any thinking and does not use the brain. It is very fast.

Pain signals are then sent via the spinal cord up to the base of the brain to an area called the *thalamus*. Here, the signals are processed again and signals are sent to the areas controlling heart rate, breathing rate, blood pressure, emotions and behaviour. The result is that you breathe faster, your heart rate and blood pressure rise, you may frown or look shocked, and you may shout 'Ow!' In addition, pain signals are sent to the outer surface of the brain (the *sensory cortex*) and an accurate picture of the type and the location of the pain is given.

Does every signal sent by the nerve to the spinal cord get sent up to the brain? No, and there are several different ways in which the way you feel pain may be influenced, one of which is the 'Gate Theory', described below.

The Gate Theory of Pain

When a nociceptor is stimulated by something harmful happening to its part of the body, an electrical message is sent to the spinal cord. Before the message can reach the brain it has to be relayed via a second nerve cell to the dorsal horn in the spinal cord; this controls which pain messages move to the brain and are felt as pain and which ones do not. This area acts as a powerful 'gatekeeper' of the pain process and the process is known as the 'gate control' theory of pain.

If you touch a hot stove and are at risk of burning your hand, your gatekeeper nerve cells will open the 'pain gate' wide to let the signals pass through quickly.

If other sensations from the skin arrive at the dorsal horn at the same time as the pain signals, they may 'interfere' with the pain signals, which are then prevented from being sent up the spinal cord to the brain. For example, when you bang your shin against a chair leg, you may reach down and rub the injury. This rubbing sends vibration signals along the nerve to the dorsal horn in the spinal cord, which prevents the pain signals from being sent on further. The 'gate' at the spinal cord level has been 'shut'. This theory of pain was first described by Melzack and Wall in 1965.

In contrast, messages that are weaker and do not indicate danger to the body, such as a little flea bite or a minor scratch, may be filtered out and not get through the pain gate or may pass slowly to the brain. You might not be aware of them at first, and your awareness of the discomfort might grow gradually rather than be felt immediately.

Pain signals must cross a gap, called a *synapse*, between each nerve on their way to the brain. How do these signals cross the gap? The first nerve cell secretes a special chemical called a *neurotransmitter*, which spreads across the gap and contacts receptor sites on the second nerve cell. The neurotransmitter causes a change to happen to the surface of the second cell and creates an electrical signal that travels along the length of the nerve cell.

The neurotransmitter either breaks down or returns to the first nerve cell. There are many different types of neurotransmitters, including *serotonin*. Scientists believe that serotonin plays a role in the release of chemicals called endorphins, which can block the transmission of pain signals across synapses and temporarily relieve pain. Opiate drugs mimic the body's natural chemicals for a similar result.

Is the pain process different in people with chronic pain? Scientists now believe it is, because of a process called *sensitization* of the dorsal horn. Continuous pain stimuli may cause nerve cells to change. More neurotransmitters may be released and the process of pain-signal transmission may alter. Nerve cells may develop a 'memory of pain', leading to heightened sensitivity to even small sensations.

Sensitization

Soon after an injury has happened, changes occur in the dorsal horn that make pain signals more likely to be transmitted to the brain – *sensitization*. Pain that was previously felt as mild becomes more severe, and something that was not painful may now be perceived as being painful. As the tissues heal, this sensitization normally disappears, but in some cases it persists and this may be why some people develop chronic pain.

Emotions

Our emotional state can influence how we feel pain. Normally the dorsal horns prevent most of the information that arrives from the receptors from travelling to the brain. This is so that the brain does not become overloaded with unimportant information – for example, the feel of our clothing on our body. Certain emotions can alter this filtering action. Extreme fear or rage can increase the level of filtering, so that even fewer messages get through. For example, a person involved in a road crash may be able to get themselves out of the wreckage and even to help others escape, becoming aware of their broken leg only once they are safe.

Other emotions such as anxiety can decrease the level of filtering so that more messages get through. For example, if you are very anxious about the dental work you are about to have, you are likely to find it more painful than someone who is more relaxed.

Endorphins and similar body chemicals called *enkephalins*, both produced in the brain and spinal cord, have the ability to block pain transmission.

Whilst the body can produce its own pain-killing substances, it can also produce too much of other substances that can cause pain. Some people may produce abnormally high levels of a chemical called *substance P.* At unusually high levels, substance P can intensify the pain messages sent to the brain, opening the pain gate. Researchers believe that people with fibromyalgia, a disease marked by chronic muscle pain and heightened pain sensitivity, may produce too much substance P.

Knowing these facts, we can see that there are four ways by which a person might hope to decrease the strength of pain felt because of their arthritis:

- Treat the disease process causing the pain by appropriate medications.

- Reduce the intensity of the pain signals coming from the nociceptor to the spinal cord by blocking the sensory nerve.

- Use the gate theory to your advantage by interfering with the passage of the pain signals from the spinal cord to the brain by using transcutaneous electrical nerve stimulation (TENS) or acupuncture.

- Address any negative emotions that may be increasing your perception of pain.

The Command Centre

How do pain messages actually turn into the pain you feel? When cells experience some type of damage – whether due to injury or to disease – the cells release chemicals into the bloodstream, such as cytokines, prostaglandins, serotonin, histamines and more. When the system works properly, the chemicals released stimulate nociceptors, which send messages via the dorsal horn of the spinal cord to the brain.

When pain messages pass through the pain gate to your brain, they first come to the brain's processing facility, the *thalamus.* The thalamus sorts and prioritizes pain messages and then sends them on to two other parts of the brain for processing: the *sensory cerebral cortex* and the *limbic centre.* It is only when the messages reach the sensory cortex that you actually *feel* pain. As we said earlier, the entire process usually happens in an instant, so you are unaware of the complicated journey of the pain messages.

DIFFERENT TYPES OF PAIN

Your doctor may use different terms to classify and describe your pain. This is important because the methods he will use to reduce and manage your pain will depend on its type. We explain the different types here.

All pain can be divided into nociceptive and non-nociceptive pain.

Nociceptive pain is initiated by the stimulation of the minute nerve receptors that are present throughout the body. It can be divided into:

- **somatic pain**, which comes from nociceptors of the the musculoskeletal system, made up of our bones, joints, muscles and skin;

- **visceral pain**, which comes from nociceptors of the the internal organs of the body, including the heart, lungs, liver, kidneys, bowels and bladder.

These types of pain usually respond to conventional pain-killers such as paracetamol, the non-steroidal anti-inflammatory drugs (NSAIDs) and opiate drugs.

Non-nociceptive pain comes from within the nervous system itself, and is caused by nerve-cell damage from trauma, nerve infection, nerve inflammation and degenerative diseases such as multiple sclerosis. It can be divided into:

- **nerve** (or **neuropathic**) **pain**, coming from the peripheral and central nervous systems;

- **sympathetic pain**, coming from the autonomic nervous system.

These types of pain respond only partly to conventional pain-killers, and other drugs are used – for example, certain antidepressants, anticonvulsants and some analgesic skin preparations. For a full discussion of all these preparations, see Chapters 4 and 5.

Nociceptive Pain

Nociceptive pain is pain sensed by the tiny nerve endings found throughout the skin and the surfaces of muscles, organs and joints. Often, nociceptive pain is caused by injuries to tissues such as muscles, ligaments, tendons, bones, joints, skin or other organs. Arthritis and an injury from a car accident are examples. Nociceptive pain often feels like aching, throbbing or a long-lasting soreness. Some doctors think that nociceptive pain, if it persists, can also cause changes in the way your nerves and spinal cord function in the pain process. If your nociceptors keep sending pain messages to the brain, you might feel pain all the time, even when there is nothing actually painful going on.

Neuropathic Pain

Pain that comes when nerves are injured or inflamed is *neuropathic pain*. This kind of pain can happen anywhere in your body, because nerves run throughout your body. Some causes of neuropathic pain are accidents or injuries, back problems that involve damaged or compressed nerves, or even nerve-damaging drugs for treating major illnesses such as cancer. Often, neuropathic pain feels like a burning sensation or a shooting pain.

Idiopathic Pain

Also called chronic pain of complex aetiology, *idiopathic pain* is a term for a painful condition of unknown cause. Doctors don't know (or don't yet know) the internal mechanisms that cause these painful problems, but the pain is very real for those who have them. They include fibromyalgia and myofascial pain. Because their doctors cannot readily identify a clear physical cause of the pain, people with these disorders often cannot find proper treatment or relief. People with this type of pain may find it difficult to communicate the nature of their pain to their doctors, creating more obstacles to pain relief. Chronic emotional stress may trigger these painful conditions in part, or it may make it worse.

LIVING WITH PAIN

Pain can have a major impact on your ability to lead a normal, fulfilling life. We're not talking about short-lived pain from a broken ankle or an ear infection. Whilst such acute pain can be severe, it lasts for a few days and can be treated effectively.

In contrast, chronic pain, like that caused by arthritis, fibromyalgia, gout, lupus, back pain, tendinitis or similar diseases, can prevent you from doing or enjoying basic activities. It can keep you from working, taking care of your home and your family, doing your daily chores or participating in hobbies and leisure activities.

Pain can be a major cause of *disability* for some people with chronic diseases such as arthritis. 'Disability' is a term that means the lack of ability to work or take care of yourself without help. People whose pain worsens to the point where they experience disability may have to apply for state benefits or depend heavily on family or loved ones for help, or both. Your doctor will work with you to determine the impact pain is having on your ability to function by measuring your pain using special charts and talking to you about what activities you can and cannot do. We talk more about these methods in Chapter 2.

ARTHRITIS: A MAJOR CAUSE OF CHRONIC PAIN

Arthritis is a major cause of chronic pain, affecting as many as 9 million people in the UK. There are over 200 kinds of arthritis, and they can affect anyone of any age. Arthritis symptoms include pain that can range from mild and occasional to severe and persistent, as well as joint swelling, fatigue and impaired movement.

Why does arthritis cause so much pain and so many problems for so many people? One reason is that arthritis is a degenerative disease – the joint damage worsens as the disease progresses – and so pain is long-lasting. Arthritis often affects other parts of the body besides joints. Because of their arthritis pain, many people stop exercising or doing much movement at all, causing their muscles to 'waste' and *atrophy,* becoming weaker. Lack of exercise can contribute to other health problems, such as obesity and cardiovascular problems, and can worsen nightly sleep, sapping energy during the day.

Of the more than 200 different forms of arthritis and related rheumatic diseases, some cause inflammation of the joints. A joint is the structure where two bones meet, and arthritis can affect joints in many parts of the body: knees, hips, back, hands, elbows, fingers, ankles. Some forms of arthritis are due to damage caused by wear and tear; others involve inflammation. In all of them, though, pain is a major feature.

Whilst many people with arthritis do not show visible signs of their disease on their bodies (although it should be visible in X-rays and other tests), some people develop deformity of joints after a period of time, deformity that usually is permanent. Other people's arthritis pain may be apparent in the way they move, or in how they restrict their activities.

Osteoarthritis

The most common form of arthritis is *osteoarthritis,* which affects about eight out of ten people over the age of 50, although it can affect younger people. People tend to develop osteoarthritis (also known as OA) as they age, when their joints start to wear down because they have been used repeatedly over many years of activity. Injuries to the joint and excessive pressure on weight-bearing joints such as the hip and knee (e.g. as that caused by being overweight) can also lead to the development of osteoarthritis, even at a relatively young age.

In osteoarthritis, the smooth, rubbery substance that protects the surfaces of the bones where they meet at a joint, called *cartilage*, breaks down. Cartilage allows the bones in the joint to move properly, so when it breaks down, bones may rub against each other, causing pain. Loose bits of cartilage may float around in the joint, causing pain and 'locking', and knobby growths called *bone spurs* may form on the bones, leading to more pain.

Each joint – consisting of bones, *tendons* (thick, cordlike tissues that connect muscles to the bones), *ligaments* (tough tissue cords that connect the bones to each other and help them move) and, sometimes, *bursae* (fluid-filled sacs that cushion the joint) – is enclosed by the joint capsule. A thin membrane called the *synovium* lines the joint capsule. The synovium secretes a slippery liquid, called *synovial fluid,* that lubricates the joint.

In osteoarthritis, the synovium can deteriorate and the volume of synovial fluid may decrease. This can make it harder for the bones in the joint to move properly, causing stiffness and more discomfort.

Rheumatoid Arthritis

Rheumatoid arthritis is a less common form of arthritis that is due to an inflammatory process. It affects between one and three people out of a hundred – mostly between between 30 and 50 years of age, but it is estimated that about 12,000 children in the UK have juvenile arthritis. RA, as it is sometimes called, is an *autoimmune disease* – a disease where the body's immune system malfunctions.

The body's disease-fighting cells secrete proteins called *antibodies.* Antibodies normally attack organisms that may enter the body, such as bacteria or viruses. In autoimmune diseases such as RA, antibodies attack parts of the body instead, and in these cases they are called *autoantibodies.* In the case of rheumatoid arthritis, these autoantibodies attack the joints and destroy the synovium, or joint lining, leading to inflammation, severe pain, stiffness and immobility. In RA, other organs of the body may also be affected in some cases. There are a number of other autoimmune diseases that have chronic pain as a major symptom, outlined later.

Fibromyalgia

Fibromyalgia is a common arthritis-related disease marked by chronic, widespread muscle pain and fatigue but does not affect the joints. About 11 per cent of the population, mostly women, are believed to have fibromyalgia, but it is difficult to estimate how many people may have the disease but are undiagnosed, so the number may be much higher.

As we learned when discussing substance P, people with fibromyalgia experience hypersensitivity to pain and feel tenderness throughout their body. Some particularly tender regions, known as *tender points*, are usually located near joints, which is a reason why people with fibromyalgia are sometimes misdiagnosed with arthritis or tendinitis. People with fibromyalgia often experience other symptoms, including difficulty sleeping, anxiety, stomach distress, changes in mood, jaw pain, headaches, irritable bowel syndrome and bladder spasms. All of these problems can worsen the person's pain.

Bursitis, Tendinitis and Similar Diseases

Bursitis, tendinitis and similar diseases known as *soft-tissue rheumatic syndromes* affect different tissues within the joints. These conditions can be very painful and can recur often. These conditions don't usually cause permanent damage, but they can affect your daily life

Bursitis is an inflammation of a bursa, a small sac located inside the joint between bone and muscle, skin or tendon. Bursae (the plural of bursa) cushion these structures.

When injury, excessive use (such as from exercise or physical activity) or calcium deposits cause the bursae to become inflamed, the result is severe pain and, sometimes, difficulty moving the affected joint. Pain usually lasts for only a few days to a few weeks, but it can flare again and again.

Tendinitis is an inflammation of a tendon, a thick fibrous cord that attaches muscles to bones in a way that allows movement at the joints. Common types of tendinitis include *rotator cuff* tendinitis (inflammation of the tendons allowing rotation at the shoulder), Achilles tendinitis (inflammation of the Achilles tendon, which is located at the back of the ankle) and de Quervain's tendinitis (inflammation of a tendon in the thumb).

There are also many common, painful disorders similar to bursitis and tendinitis, including *carpal tunnel syndrome*. A painful and sometimes debilitating disorder, carpal tunnel syndrome is caused by pressure on the median nerve in the wrist, which produces pain, numbness, swelling, weakness and thumb mobility problems. Sometimes, both wrists are affected.

Causes of carpal tunnel syndrome include repetitive use, such as in typing long hours at a computer keyboard, something millions of people do every day. Other diseases, such as thyroid gland conditions, diabetes, infection, rheumatoid arthritis or other types of inflammatory arthritis, can also lead to carpal tunnel syndrome. A small percentage of people with carpal tunnel syndrome require surgery to correct the problem and restore normal hand ability. Usually, identifying the cause and taking anti-inflammatory medications will ease their painful symptoms.

The type of nerve compression found in carpal tunnel syndrome can also occur in the ankles, a condition called *tarsal tunnel syndrome.* Tarsal tunnel syndrome causes painful, burning sensations in the foot, the sole or the toes.

Another painful condition affecting the soft tissues in the joints is *lateral epicondylitis*, commonly known as *tennis elbow.* Whilst you don't have to play tennis to have tennis elbow, the condition is common among people who play similar sports or do strenuous gardening using their arms. Any repetitive action that lifts the wrists may cause tennis elbow. It's an inflammation of the *lateral epicondyle,* an area of the bone where the muscles are attached to the outer elbow.

Tennis elbow is a painful condition that involves an aching, persistent pain from the outside of the elbow down the forearm. Basic activities, including moving the fingers, lifting an object with the hand and wrist, turning a doorknob or opening a jar, can become painful and difficult.

When the inside of the elbow is affected, this is called *medial epicondylitis*, or *golfer's elbow.* Overusing the muscles used for flexing the wrist can cause golfer's elbow, which gives pain in the inner part of the elbow or pain in the fingers or wrists when bending them.

Other soft tissues can become inflamed or pressured from excessive use, causing pain, swelling and other symptoms. One such con-

dition – called *stenosing tenosynovitis* or *trigger finger* – stems from a thickening of the lining around the tendons in the fingers, causing the finger to lock in a painful, bent position and then to snap open suddenly. Trigger finger can cause tenderness, swelling or small bumps in the palm, and aching pain in the middle joint of the affected finger.

Similarly, the thick, fibrous tissue stretching across the sole of your foot, from the heel to the toes, can become inflamed, a condition called *plantar fasciitis.* Plantar fasciitis, which can result from running, excessive standing, being overweight or even having 'flat feet' or heel spurs, can cause pain in the sole (particularly in the heel) during walking.

Other Forms of Arthritis

There are many other forms of arthritis and arthritis-related diseases that involve pain that is either chronic or recurring.

- **Gout.** Gout develops because of an accumulation of a substance known as *uric acid* in the body. Gout can occur either because there is too much uric acid produced (such as from eating foods rich in *purines,* nutrients whose end-product is uric acid) or because the kidneys don't eliminate the uric acid properly, causing it to build up, crystallize and settle in joints. The primary joints affected by this crystalline build-up are those of the hands and feet. An attack of gout can be horribly painful as the build-up presses against sensitive parts of the joint and can cause inflammation.

- **Ankylosing Spondylitis.** Ankylosing spondylitis, or AS, is one of a group of arthritis-related diseases that primarily affect the joints of the spine. In ankylosing spondylitis, these joints can become inflamed, and, eventually, the tissues supporting the spine can stiffen. The person's spine can become rigid, leading to stiffness, pain and even difficulty breathing.

- **Lupus.** Lupus, short for systemic lupus erythematosus (SLE), is another auto-immune disease that leads not only to joint swelling and pain but also to skin rashes, internal organ damage and other serious problems. Lupus, like rheumatoid arthritis, occurs when the body's immune system, which should defend against disease-causing bacteria and viruses, turns on the body's tissues instead.

- **Sjögren's syndrome.** Sjögren's syndrome is another autoimmune disease that can cause inflammation of the joints and arthritis. It also causes dry eyes and mouth, and inflammation of the skin, lungs, kidneys and thyroid gland.

- **Psoriatic arthritis.** Psoriasis, a skin disease, can also cause arthritis after a number of years.

- **Reactive arthritis.** Reactive arthritis occurs in conditions in which the immune system is suppressed. These include infection, diabetes and liver disease.

- **Back Pain.** There are many ailments that fall under the umbrella of back pain, a very common health problem. There are many different possible causes for back pain. People may experience osteoarthritis in their back, causing pain and stiffness. Back pain can also be the result of muscle injuries or spasms, strains to the discs cushioning the spine's joints (at the *vertebrae*), compressed nerves or other problems. In *sciatica* there is pain that travels across the buttock and down the leg, sometimes as far as the foot. It's caused when the sciatic nerve, which runs from your spinal cord down your legs to your feet, is put under pressure or irritated. Back pain can be very intense and debilitating, or nagging and mild.

There are many other forms of arthritis and related conditions, some of which you may have experienced. There are also other types of chronic pain not associated with joints or bones. Many people suffer from chronic headaches, including debilitating migraine headaches, and many people also experience chronic pain related to sports injuries or cancer. No matter what the source of your pain, many of the strategies outlined in this book may help you find relief. Whether you have osteoarthritis, fibromyalgia, bursitis, nerve pain or a herniated disc in your spine, your pain is real. Your pain affects your well-being and happiness. Your pain interferes with your ability to live your life normally.

That's why it is so important for you to explain your pain to your doctor and find the appropriate treatments for it. Communicating what is wrong is the all-important first step in

CHILDREN AND PAIN

Many children also have chronic conditions that cause serious pain, including some form of juvenile arthritis or a related disease.

Arthritis affects one child in 1,000 in the UK. There is no known cause of this disease, which is different from arthritis in adults.

Fortunately, most children with arthritis will lead full and active lives. Moreover, the problems associated with the condition are not generally long-lasting.

The right medicines and exercises will make a great difference, and better medicines and treatments are being developed.

The best way forward for a child with arthritis is to involve the entire family in the treatment.

Organizations that offer help include:

- **Arthritis Care**: services include a helpline, information days, a magazine and the booklets *A Day with Sam* and *Chat 2 Parents: arthritis in teenagers*

- **Arthritis Research Campaign**: services include the booklets *Arthritis in Teenagers* and *Tim has Arthritis*

- **Children's Chronic Arthritis Association**

- **Choices**: services include the booklet *Kids with Arthritis: a guide for parents*

- **JOINTZ** (Arthritis Care's support group for parents in Northern Ireland): which has a video *Physio for Kids*

Contact details of these organizations are in the Resources section.

---

finding a solution. Yet, in some cases, this step can be the most difficult. Sometimes it's hard to describe just how and where it hurts. In this chapter, we show you some ways to do this effectively.

Are All Pains Equal?

Obviously, all pains are not equal. Although two people may have the same disease or condition, their pain may be different, and the way they perceive and react to their pain may also differ.

Pain comes in different forms: aches, burns, stings, throbs, tingles, stabs, and on and on. The pain from stubbing your toe on the filing cabinet in the office will feel very different from the pain of stepping on a nail when you're barefoot at the beach. More severe pain will elicit a much stronger chemical response from the brain: you will feel the pain faster and more intensely.

Pain can ebb and flow. Your pain may seem worse at certain times than at others. A knee with arthritis may feel worse after you have been walking around the shops, for example. Pain often feels worse at night when there is little or nothing to distract you. Your physical makeup, background, emotional state, the pain you have experienced in the past and other personal factors affect how you sense pain and react to it. If your pain is chronic rather than acute, the repeated pain messages sent to the brain might alter your perception of the pain.

Let's say you and a friend are going together to donate blood. You have never donated blood before, and you are nervous about the process. When the technician inserts the needle into the vein in your arm to draw the blood, you might find the insertion uncomfortable or painful. It may even make you feel anxious. But your friend, who has donated blood many times before and has no anxiety about the process, only 'feels' a slight sting. The action is the same, but the person's unique makeup creates different sensations.

Explaining About Your Pain

It's important for you to find ways to explain the intensity and the nature of your pain to your doctor. Doctors have many tools to help you describe and identify your pain.

Your consultation will include a medical history, during which your doctor or a nurse will ask you questions about your current and past medical problems and what medications you may have taken. The medical history may also include various questionnaires to determine the nature of your problem and the underlying cause of your pain. Your doctor

will perform a clinical examination, and may then arrange a number of laboratory tests and X-rays. By pinpointing its type and cause, your doctor will be able to prescribe the right medications and suggest the appropriate measures to address your pain.

In some cases, medical tests and questions may not immediately reveal the cause of your pain or an appropriate course of action. It's important for you to stay optimistic! Whilst you may have to learn to deal with certain amounts of pain in your life, pain should not become so overwhelming that you have to stay in bed for a week or not be able to walk to the postbox. You and your doctor should continue to try various methods for treating your pain.

If necessary, you may be referred by your GP to a specialist, a doctor with additional training in a particular medical field. If you have arthritis that is causing more than mild, occasional pain and stiffness, you might see a rheumatologist – a doctor who has additional training in diagnosing and treating arthritis and related rheumatic diseases (such as those described earlier in this chapter). Or your pain may become so intense that you require surgical treatment from an *orthopaedic surgeon,* a doctor who specializes in surgery of the bones and joints.

If you have chronic, debilitating pain and need special, ongoing treatment for it, you might see a pain specialist, who is usually an *anaesthetist* who specializes in pain medicine. These doctors, rather than administering anaesthesia for surgery (which numbs you or makes you sleep while the operation is happening), can help treat your pain and administer various pain treatments that we discuss in this book.

Finding Ways to Fight Pain

Pain, as we said earlier, is a unique experience for each person. Some people may have mild chronic pain that becomes bothersome only on an occasional basis. Other people may have intense pain that interferes with their ability to work and live a normal life.

It's up to you to determine what is tolerable for you. Together with your doctor, you should be able to find some strategies that relieve your pain. You should not have to 'grin and bear it' when there are many treatments that can control pain.

Some people worry about the *side effects* of painkillers or other drugs. These effects, which can range from stomach disorders to constipation to grogginess, are a real concern for many people. Some drugs can have dangerous side effects, so it's important for you to let your doctor know immediately if you develop any new or troublesome symptom.

Your doctor should be able to work with you to find the right drugs, or combination of drugs if necessary, and the proper dosage of each drug to give you the maximum benefit with the least side effects. If side effects are becoming a health hazard of their own, let your doctor know. You may have to switch drugs, lower the dosage you take, or try other methods of relieving your pain. In Chapter 3 we outline some ways to deal with side effects of common drugs.

Not all pain-control strategies involve drugs or other medical treatments. There are many other ways to relieve pain. We learn about many of these methods in this book. Exercise, diet, complementary therapies such as *acupuncture* or *herbal supplements*, movement techniques such as *yoga, t'ai chi* or the *Alexander technique* can also help you alleviate your pain. Relaxation techniques can reduce your stress, easing pain by relaxing tense muscles. These other therapies can augment medical treatments and be very effective.

One of the most powerful weapons you have in the battle against pain is your mind. Your brain is the centre of pain perception, as well as the centre of emotions that govern how you respond to pain. Your brain also contains great power to deal with pain and even to lessen pain. In this book you will learn strategies to harness your mind's power to fight pain, including *guided imagery* and *meditation.* With these methods and more, you may be able to close that pain gate so that pain does not take over your life.

In the next chapter, we look at how your doctor will diagnose the cause of your pain and take the first steps in recommending treatments.

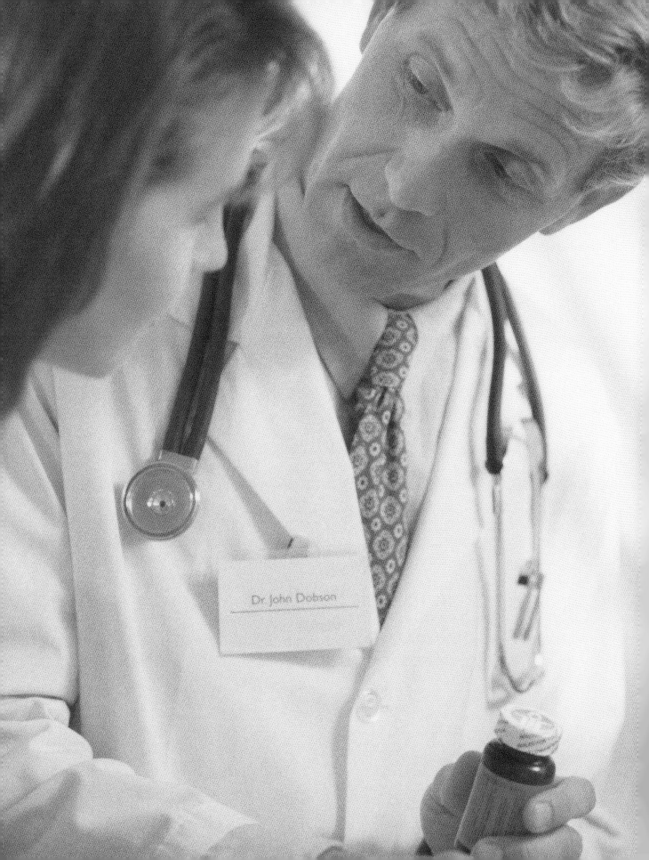

Dr. John Dobson

What's Causing
Your Pain?

2

CHAPTER 2: WHAT'S CAUSING YOUR PAIN?

When you have serious, chronic pain that doesn't go away with over-the-counter treatments or rest, your first action should be to pick up the phone and make an appointment with your GP. Your second action should be – in partnership with your GP – doing what it takes to find the cause of your pain. When you know what causes your pain, you can move to the third step: creating a comprehensive pain-management plan that works.

Other than its origins and its duration, how does chronic pain differ from acute pain? Chronic pain – such as the pain of arthritis, fibromyalgia, nerve damage, spinal cord injuries, or other serious diseases such as cancer – involves a process slightly different from that for acute pain.

In acute pain, such as that from an injury, the nerve endings that sense pain (the nociceptors) send a signal to the dorsal horn of the spinal cord. Usually this message is sent on up to the brain, where the sensation of pain is perceived. Powerful drugs, for example opiates such as codeine, can be used on a short-term basis to relieve severe pain of short duration.

Chronic pain may be more complex to treat. Because the problems causing the pain are present over a long period of time, pain-sensing nerves can become even more sensitive to the stimulus. Some researchers believe that repeated stimulation might cause these nerves to send continuous pain signals to the brain even when the pain-causing condition has been treated or resolved.

So treating chronic pain can be challenging for doctors and patients alike. Many people do not like the prospect of taking pain-killing drugs on a regular, long-term basis. However, there are new types of drugs and other treatments that may lessen chronic pain effectively with fewer side effects than from some of the older drugs.

FINDING THE CAUSE OF YOUR PAIN

As we learned in Chapter 1, you and your doctor are not just treating the pain. You are searching for the disease or problem that is causing the pain. Treatments may address the cause of the disease – such as rheumatoid arthritis or gout as well as treating the pain it causes.

If you have rheumatoid arthritis, for example, your doctor might prescribe a *corticosteroid* medication such as prednisolone, or another *disease-modifying antirheumatic drug*, such as methotrexate, to address the inflammation or the immune system malfunction that is causing your joints to swell and hurt. You may also need treatments, perhaps both medical and complementary, to relieve the pain caused by the disease.

Before you can begin to discuss treating your pain, you and your doctor must try to pinpoint pain's cause. To do this, you have to find an effective way of communicating the nature and intensity of your pain to your doctor and other members of the health-care team. It's vital that you make the most of the short time you may have to talk to your doctor about your pain and related symptoms so that you can find an effective treatment for your pain as soon as possible.

In this chapter, we discuss techniques your doctor may use to diagnose the cause of your pain, and we explain further the main causes of chronic pain that you may be experiencing. We also show you ways to communicate more effectively and efficiently with your doctor and his or her staff.

Diagnosis: Tests and Questions

Diagnosis is the first and most important step in pain treatment. The word 'diagnosis' comes from the Greek word meaning 'to distinguish', and the process of diagnosis involves learning more about your problem by looking at all the facts about your health. Like a detective, your doctor and members of staff will ask you various questions and perform tests, if necessary, to gather information about you and your health.

During your first appointment, your doctor will probably take the following steps to form a diagnosis:

• Take a *medical history*, asking you about your present and past health problems, medical procedures or injuries, and health problems that your close family members may have had.

• Discuss all the medications and other therapies you have used (not only for pain, but for other health problems as well).

• Use some type of pain assessment test, such as a pain scale or questionnaire, or just talk to you about your pain.

• Conduct a through *physical examination.*

• *Test* blood, urine or other bodily fluids.

• In some instances, conduct tests such as X-rays, magnetic resonance imaging (MRI), computed axial tomography (CAT or CT) scans, dual X-ray absorptiometry (DEXA) scans and others to examine bones and soft tissues.

These techniques and tests will help your doctor determine the probable cause of your pain and to assess joint damage or other problems that may already have occurred. These facts will help your doctor decide what steps to take to treat your pain.

Describing your pain is the most important first step in treatment. Your doctor might talk to you or give you tests designed to gather and quantify data about your pain. Answer these questions as accurately as possible. Try not to exaggerate or minimize any problems you have. If possible, before your appointment with your doctor, write down a basic description of your problems and a timeline of when and how they occurred. Also have a brief medical history ready if you have not discussed this with your doctor before. See p. 31 for more information about your medical history.

Members of Your Health-Care Team

At some point you may be referred by your GP to another health professional, including a specialist at your local hospital, to help you manage the various aspects of your disease. In addition to a rheumatologist or an orthopaedic surgeon, the people who may be part of your health-care team include the following professionals.

Other doctors. Because different forms of arthritis can be systemic, meaning that they affect the entire body, your care may involve seeing doctors who specialize in treating organs and systems affected by arthritis-related disease. In addition to rheumatologists and orthopaedic surgeons, these doctors may include dermatologists, who specialize in treating problems of the skin, hair and nails; ophthalmologists, who specialize in problems of the eyes; nephrologists, who specialize in kidney disease; geriatricians, who specialize in the treatment of older people; and paediatric rheumatologists, who specialize in treating arthritis in children.

Not all of the therapists will necessarily be available to you through the NHS – for example, massage therapists or acupuncturists. Moreover, some NHS services, such as chiropody/podiatry, can be in short supply, resulting in a long wait to be seen.

Physiotherapist. If arthritis causes pain and limited motion in your joints, or causes difficulties with walking, stretching, bending or climbing stairs, a physiotherapist (physio) may help. A physio can devise an exercise plan that strengthens your muscles and increases your range of motion. Physios also prescribe such devices as canes, splints or shoe inserts. Many physios are trained in soft-tissue massage, which people with arthritis often find helpful to relieve pain and stiffness.

Occupational therapist. An occupational therapist (OT) can help you find ways to manage daily tasks at home and at work. If arthritis makes it difficult to do such tasks as cooking, typing, driving, brushing your teeth or buttoning your clothes, an OT may suggest different ways to do these tasks or arrange for 'assistive' devices or splints.

Nurses. In addition to taking your blood pressure, drawing blood and providing routine care, nurses function as patient educators and advocates. When you visit your GP practice or health centre, you might well be seen by a practice nurse for routine matters. Practice nurses work alongside GPs, giving the GPs time to concentrate on more complex medical matters. A role being developed for experienced nurses is that of nurse practitioner; nurse practitioners will be trained further to help doctors in diagnosis, evaluating and monitoring patients, and in some cases writing prescriptions and carrying out minor surgery as well.

State registered dietitian. Diet and weight management are important in arthritis,

WORKING WITH YOUR DOCTOR: FINDING THE RIGHT FIT

Managing your arthritis requires a team effort. But what if your doctor doesn't want you to be a part of the team? Many doctors appreciate informed, involved patients, but there are exceptions.

Some doctors view a patient's questions as a sign of distrust or are put off by patients who want to take charge of their own health care. For some patients, such doctors are fine. Just as there are doctors who want you to follow their orders – full stop – there are patients who prefer to put all of their medical decisions in the hands of the doctor. These patients find comfort in knowing that someone else is in charge.

Although the best doctor–patient relationship is one in which there is some give-and-take, what's most important is that you see eye-to-eye with your doctor.

Problems can arise when there is a discrepancy between the way you and your doctor prefer to work. If you want to take a role in your health care, but your doctor expects you to follow orders without question, it may be time to find a new doctor.

Before you switch, however, be sure that you're not asking for or expecting too much. Although your doctor should be willing to answer questions and be open to the possibility of different treatments you would like to try, no doctor has the time to answer endless lists of queries from every patient.

A doctor who merely agrees with everything you suggest is not good for you. And prescribing or condoning every treatment you mention can be downright dangerous.

---

because excess weight can add stress to fragile joints and can complicate joint surgery. A proper diet can help you reduce your risk of other health problems, such as diabetes, cardiovascular disease and some cancers. A consultation with a dietitian may help you find a healthy diet that fits your lifestyle.

Psychologist. When you're struggling with a chronic disease, it's understandable that you may get depressed. Mental-health professionals can help you deal with the psychological aspects of your illness, such as depression, anxiety and anger.

Psychologists cannot prescribe medications. If you have a problem that requires or would be helped by medication, they will refer you to a psychiatrist. Psychiatrists are medical doctors with psychiatric training who can prescribe such medications as antidepressants.

Pharmacist. No matter which type of arthritis you have, there is a good chance that you will take some type of medication for it. Your pharmacist can be a good source of information about the medications your doctor prescribes and the medications you purchase over the counter (i.e. without a prescription). Don't hesitate to ask your pharmacist questions about side effects, how to take medication or which sorts of over-the-counter medications are appropriate for you.

Podiatrist and chiropodist. A podiatrist, or chiropodist, treats conditions of the foot, from nail infections to arthritis-damaged joints. Podiatrists are licensed to perform minor surgery. If arthritis affects your feet, a podiatrist may be a member of your healthcare team.

Dentist. If Sjögren's syndrome causes dry mouth, if arthritis affects your jaw joint (a condition called temporomandibular joint disorder) or makes it difficult to perform proper oral hygiene, you're particularly vulnerable to dental problems. For that reason, it's especially important that you see a dentist regularly to detect and take care of any problems before they become severe. In addition, a dentist may offer advice on how to brush and floss your teeth if arthritis affects your hands.

Acupuncturist. If you need help with pain and are willing to try complementary therapy, you may want to see an acupuncturist. Acupuncturists insert slender needles into the skin at various points on the body to relieve pain. The theory behind acupuncture is that the practice corrects the flow of qi, the body's vital energy, which optimizes health. Modern research suggests that acupuncture may ease pain by causing the release of endorphins. A few acupuncturists are also doctors. Check an acupuncturist's credentials before you make your first appointment. Nowadays, some physiotherapists can perform acupuncture as well.

Massage therapist. You know how good it feels to have your back and shoulders rubbed when you are achy and stiff. Massage therapists are specially trained and certified to perform therapeutic massage, which can relieve muscle tension, improve range of motion and, perhaps, ease pain. You might also receive massage from a physio.

Chiropractor. Chiropractors use manual manipulation of the joints to increase range of motion and help relieve pain.

For people with certain types of arthritis, however, manipulations may not be indicated or safe. Chiropractors do not perform surgery or prescribe medication.

What If You Don't Have a Doctor?

You may be in pain – but what if you don't know whom to call for help?

Not everyone has an established relationship with a general practitioner (GP). There are many reasons why you may not have a doctor to turn to. You may have moved home and don't know the doctors in your new neighbourhood. Your previous doctor may have retired. Or, until now, you never felt the need to go to a doctor. But now you do. What do you do?

Whether or not a person has a chronic illness or any illness at all, it's important to have some kind of ongoing, regular care from a GP. The GP will monitor your overall health and address problems as needed. When you feel ill or become injured, you will be able to turn to a professional who understands your particular situation and past medical problems.

If you are experiencing chronic pain, it's very important to have a regular relationship with a doctor. It's likely that you will need ongoing care for your health problem and periodic visits to monitor treatment and progress.

Your local library should have a list of doctors in your area, or contact your Primary Care Trust for help in finding a GP.

Choosing your doctor. A number of factors will help you decide which doctors are good candidates to become *your* doctor:

- The location of the practice: is it convenient?

- Is the doctor's gender or age important to you?

- The doctor's experience and training: do you feel confident in his ability?

- The experiences of other patients: do they speak well of him, his staff and his services?

- The time the doctor usually spends with a patient: is there enough time to discuss your problems? Can you book a double appointment?

When you narrow your choices, you may wish to ask the doctor or his staff the following important questions:

- Does this doctor or practice accept new patients at this time?

- What are the days of the week and hours that the office is open for appointments?

- Typically, how much advance notice is needed to make appointments?

- On average, how long does the doctor spend with each patient? What about support staff?

- If I have an emergency, how quickly can I arrange an appointment?

- What can I do if I have a medical problem after hours or when the doctor is on holiday?

Remember: Your choice of doctor is important. If you are not satisfied, you can always seek the services of another doctor. Speak frankly to your doctor about your needs and concerns. Chances are, your doctor wishes to make you feel well treated as well as to treat your health problems.

Pain Clinics

Your primary-care doctor (your GP) may diagnose the cause of your pain and begin the treatment process. If you don't get adequate pain relief from the treatments your doctor suggests, he can, if necessary, refer you to a pain specialist. These doctors may have various medical backgrounds, but many are anaesthetists with additional training in pain-management. You may associate anaesthetists with surgery, and these doctors do work in surgical settings to anaesthetize the patient during the procedure (so he or she doesn't feel the pain of the operation). However, some anaesthetists specialize in treating ongoing pain and offer helpful treatments and long-term pain-management techniques.

Pain specialists work in hospitals and focus only on pain management. These special facilities are called *pain clinics*. In a pain clinic doctors of various specialties and other health-care professionals work together to address a wide variety of chronic pain problems. Each doctor has a different area of expertise, and all can consult together on patients in pain. The pain clinic probably has nurses, physiotherapists, occupational therapists and psychologists on its staff to help you adapt to your pain or deal with the emotional impact of chronic pain.

Pain clinics, which are usually in large hospital complexes, might also have other professionals available to advise you about other areas of your life. These professionals might include counsellors, social workers and dietitians, or even a chaplain. Pain affects your whole life, including your job and your personal relationships. These professionals may help you adjust to your chronic pain, or help you find ways to make positive improvements to your health (such as to lose excess weight) to increase pain relief.

When you go to a pain clinic, the pain specialist will probably repeat some of the basic testing that your primary-care doctor conducted. You can expect to discuss your medical history, have a physical examination and perhaps undergo some diagnostic tests (such as X-rays). These steps allow the doctor to confirm your diagnosis and suggest possible treatment.

Then, the doctor will discuss the pros and cons of the available treatments. Once you decide together how to proceed, your treatment begins. If you don't achieve adequate relief, your doctor will try other treatments to continue the search for a solution.

If you don't have a pain clinic in your area, it's very likely that your primary-care doctor can administer the pain-relief methods described in this chapter, or refer you to a specialist who can. If necessary, you may have to travel some distance to see a pain specialist. Make arrangements with a friend or family member to accompany you to these sessions if possible.

What happens if you don't find a medical treatment that relieves your pain? Your pain specialist may be able to help you learn how to adapt to your new situation, difficult as it may be. These pain-management programmes allow you to learn ways to modify your activities, use non-medical techniques to relax or cope with the stress of chronic pain, find a support network of friends or family members to help you handle daily tasks, and try various non-drug or even complementary pain-relief techniques to help you manage your pain.

There is more about pain-management on p. 43.

The first step in any doctor's or health-care professional's management will be to get some background information on you, your painful condition and your general health state. To begin, he or she will probably take a medical history.

What Is Your Medical History?

A medical history is the story of your health. This story includes chapters about illnesses, injuries or health problems you have now or have had in the past; your record of vaccinations; allergies; any health conditions or medical problems your close family members have had; and medications or treatments you have used, and any side effects they may have caused. These pieces of information come together to a form your 'health profile', often revealing where you may be at risk for developing certain diseases or problems. Also, your medical history suggests what treatments may or may not be effective for you.

When you make your first appointment with a new doctor, you may be asked to fill out some forms prior to your visit, about your medical history, current state of health and other important facts. Your doctor will then go over your medical history face to face during your consultation. They will keep a record of this information so they can refer to it on future visits.

However, it may be helpful for you to write down your own medical history before you go to your appointment. By doing this, you will be able to remember problems you may have had long ago, and you will have the opportunity to contact relatives if you have questions about diseases that may be common in your family.

Spend an hour or so writing down what medical problems you have had during your lifetime. Include major injuries or illnesses, such as a car accident, recurring episodes of back pain, a broken bone that required medical care, pneumonia or chickenpox. List what immunizations you have had, and check past medical records for this information if you have them. Try to recall if you have ever had any unusual test results in your blood, urine, blood pressure, heartbeat or reflexes. Have you ever been told that you have high blood pressure? Have you gained or lost a great deal of weight in the past? Have you had surgery for any reason?

In addition, what sort of examinations or tests have you had in the past – such as a blood test, mammogram, cervical smear, prostate examination or colonoscopy – and what were the results? Your doctor can request important test results from your past doctors if necessary. It's important to note if you or your parents, grandparents or siblings ever had any major illnesses or health problems, including:

• Diabetes

• Stroke

• Heart attack or heart problems

• Cancer

- Arthritis or a related disease

- Osteoporosis

- Gastrointestinal diseases

- Alcoholism or drug abuse

- High blood pressure

- Depression

- Other major health problems

If your parents or grandparents had some diseases or health problems, you may be more at risk for developing them. This doesn't mean that you are certain to get this illness – it just means that you should be aware of the warning signs, and make lifestyle changes if necessary. Your doctor will ask follow-up questions if he needs to know more about your medical past. These facts all blend together to create your health profile. Using this profile, your doctor will be able to address any problems and monitor your ongoing health care.

Talking to Your Doctor About Pain

Before you see the doctor, a nurse may perform a few basic tests to assess your current physical condition. The nurse may weigh and measure you; take your blood pressure; and ask you to urinate in a small cup to test your urine.

Don't be frustrated by these tests: they're necessary to get a clearer picture of your situation. Even though these tests may not relate specifically to your pain, they will help your doctor assess your overall health. Your health may have an impact on your pain whether you realize it or not. For example, if you are overweight for your height and age, the excess pounds may be putting too much stress on your hips and knees. If you have arthritis in your hips or knees, this might make the pain worse.

The doctor will now ask you some questions about your pain and related symptoms. It's important to communicate your problems effectively to the doctor because he may not have a great deal of time to spend with you. So make the most of that time! If you prepare a bit before your appointment, you'll be one step ahead in the process.

As we suggested you do with your medical history, sit down for a little while before your appointment to think about your pain. Create a summary of your condition by writing informal notes about what you are feeling. Ask yourself the following questions to help you form your summary:

- **How does the pain feel?** Try to find words that describe the actual sensation, such as burning, aching, tingling, stinging, etc.

- **Where does the pain occur in the body?** Be as specific as possible. For instance, does your leg hurt? At the thigh, the hip, the knee or the ankle?

- **When does pain occur?** Does pain worsen at certain times of day, such as late afternoon after you have been sitting at your desk all day, or in connection with certain activities, such as after you exercise?

- **Do you experience other symptoms on a regular basis?** Note anything that seems unusual, such as stomach pain, nausea, fatigue, inability to fall asleep, headaches, pain with sexual activity, etc. Do these symptoms seem to occur in connection with your pain?

- **How long have you been experiencing this pain?** Did it start suddenly, or did you notice it gradually?

- **How intense is the pain?** Is it mild but annoying? Or is it so intense at times that you cannot function, sleep, move your joint, have sex, or perform other daily, necessary activities? Pain intensity may be difficult to describe to your doctor. Your doctor can offer you some helpful mechanisms for doing so.

- **What makes it worse?** Perhaps keep a diary in which you note bad periods, to see if there is a pattern.

- **Does anything make it better?** Does it always help or only sometimes? How? When?

How to Describe Pain

Pain is a personal experience that is very difficult to describe to others. Two people with very similar conditions may perceive their pain differently. Many factors may affect how you feel and react to pain: for example, personal history, personality, cultural makeup, gender, age.

Arthritis pain is also very subjective. Arthritis can involve many different symp-toms, affect different joints and organs, and manifest distinctly from one person to the next. One standard of arthritis pain is that it is chronic. However, each person may find that the pain worsens at some times and lessens at others.

It's important for you to work out the patterns in your pain and what factors may trigger or alleviate your pain, and to communicate this information to your doctor. To understand your pain, your doctor may use various tools to help assess or quantify that pain. These tools include:

- **Pain scales,** which are charts designed to help you rate the intensity of your pain. For example, you might rate the pain you experience on a scale of 1 to 10, where 1 is having no pain and 10 is the worst pain imaginable. Your pain might vary in intensity depending on certain factors, and this scale would help you explain to your doctor the variance between times when your pain is tolerable and times when your pain flares or gets suddenly worse.

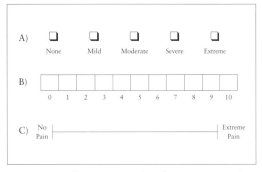

QUANTIFYING PAIN: Examples of various pain scales.

- **Pain questionnaires,** which are a series of questions about your pain, where it is located, what words or comparisons you can use to describe it, what makes it worse, and other factors. For example, you might feel 'burning' in your left hip that gets worse after you have been on your feet all day at work, or a 'dull ache' and 'stiffness' in your knees that is worst in the morning and gets better after your shower. There are many different types of pain questionnaires, but these tools allow you to explain important facts about your pain so that your doctor can evaluate the nature of your problem. A complete example of an actual pain questionnaire used by pain specialists is given at the end of this chapter.

- **Pain diaries** are another way for you to track your pain over a period of time. Your doctor might ask you to keep a diary for several days or weeks before your next appointment, noting when pain occurs, what parts of the body are affected by pain, the nature or intensity of the pain, and other important points. Pain diaries allow your doctor to note patterns in your pain, what factors may cause pain flares, what other symptoms may accompany your pain, and what treatments may have worked or not worked to alleviate your pain.

All of the tools used to assess your pain, and the information they provide, help your doctor diagnose the cause of the pain and determine treatment options. Different treatments might work better than others depending on the cause of your pain, your lifestyle, what treatments have worked in the past, and other factors.

PHYSICAL EXAMINATIONS AND MEDICAL TESTS

During the physical examination, your doctor may look at the joint or joints where your pain occurs, and may ask you to move the affected area. He may look for swelling, stiffness, redness or other obvious symptoms in and around the joint that point to the cause of your pain.

Your doctor may also check other parts of your body, such as the skin, eyes or mouth, to determine if you have evidence of certain illnesses that affect these organs. These signs can tell your doctor that you have certain forms of arthritis, or rule these diseases out as the cause of your chronic pain. The doctor might also ask you to walk, sit or bend to observe your gait, the curvature of your spine, the height of your shoulders and so on.

If your pain and other symptoms suggest you might have fibromyalgia, your doctor will perform a *tender point examination*. Diagnosing fibromyalgia is often imprecise and time-consuming, as medical research has not yet confirmed its true cause. However, criteria have been developed to help in making the diagnosis. These criteria help doctors rule out other problems and confirm a diagnosis of fibromyalgia.

People with fibromyalgia do not have swelling, pain or stiffness in joints themselves, as seen in arthritis. Instead, they have pain

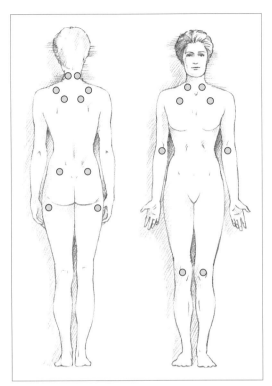

TENDER POINTS: Points of the body where fibromyalgia pain is most common

and, often, extreme tenderness or sensitivity in certain areas of the body. These areas are known as *tender points*. A person with fibromyalgia must have pain and sensitivity in at least 11 of the 18 recognized tender points. During a tender point examination, the doctor applies pressure to the 18 points and counts the number of sites where unusual pain and sensitivity occur. The chart on this page shows the 18 recognized tender points of fibromyalgia.

In order to diagnose the cause of your chronic pain, your doctor may request a variety of medical tests. The results of these tests may rule out certain ailments as well as suggest them; they may also suggest other possible ailments. We mentioned a few of these types of tests above, but here we go into a little more detail about common tests used to diagnose arthritis and related diseases. With fibromyalgia, the only reliable test at this time is the tender point examination and a verbal discussion of symptoms. But for other diseases that can cause chronic pain, body fluid and imaging tests can aid in diagnosis.

Laboratory Tests

Your blood, urine and other fluids can hold clues to the cause of your pain. For example, if tests reveal that you have abnormally high or low levels of certain chemicals in your body fluids, they might suggest the existence of certain diseases. That's why it's important for your doctor to take a urine sample and/or a small blood sample.

Here is a rundown of some common tests used to diagnose arthritis and related diseases, the chief causes of chronic pain:

Anti-DNA test. The anti-DNA blood test detects the presence of autoantibodies in the blood. Antibodies are substances made by the body that normally attach to disease-causing foreign organisms such as viruses or bacteria and help the body defend itself against their attack. Sometimes, antibodies mistakenly attack one's own DNA (the material found in the nucleus of each human cell that serves as the basic building block of life). The presence of these autoantibodies (or antibodies that attack self) is a common sign of systematic lupus erythematosus, or 'lupus' for short.

Anti-nuclear antibody test. Also known as an ANA test, this blood test reveals the existence of antibodies that mistakenly attack the nuclei (command centres) of cells, leading to cell damage. A positive result may be evidence of an autoimmune disease. ANA tests are used in diagnosis of lupus, rheumatoid arthritis, scleroderma (an arthritis-related disease involving skin damage), polymyositis (an inflammatory disease affecting muscle) and others.

Complement test. This blood test measures the level of complement, a substance that aids the body's own immune system, our defence against disease. Complement helps antibodies do their job in fighting foreign agents, such as bacteria and viruses. When levels of complement are too low, this may indicate that the person has an autoimmune disease such as vasculitis (a term for diseases marked by inflammation of the blood vessels) or lupus.

C-Reactive protein test. C-reactive protein (or CRP) is a plasma protein found in the blood. High levels of this protein are an indicator of inflammation, and can be seen in cases of infection, physical trauma, burns, advanced stages of cancer, surgery and inflammatory diseases. The CRP test is used commonly in the process of diagnosing rheumatoid arthritis and other diseases marked by inflammation. Raised levels of

CRP alone is not a sure sign of any one condition, but this test can help the doctor determine a diagnosis along with other methods.

Erythrocyte sedimentation rate (ESR) test. The ESR blood test measures how far red blood cells fall to the bottom of a test tube within a specific time. Substances in the blood that cause inflammation make red blood cells clump together. Because these heavy clumps fall faster than single red blood cells, a high ESR can indicate inflammation in the body. This test may help to diagnose rheumatoid arthritis, ankylosing spondylitis, polymyalgia rheumatica and other arthritis-related diseases that have painful inflammation as a symptom.

Full blood count test (FBC). Full blood count testing measures various components in the blood, which can be indicators of certain types of diseases. A reduced number or size or concentration of red blood cells, a condition known as *anaemia,* could indicate rheumatoid arthritis, lupus, polymyalgia rheumatica, inflammatory bowel disease or other diseases. A low count of white blood cells (which help fight disease) or platelets might indicate lupus. A high count of white blood cells might indicate an infection.

Joint fluid examination. In a joint fluid examination, the doctor withdraws fluid from the joint, which can then be tested for the presence of certain chemicals or elements. This test can help diagnose diseases such as gout, because uric acid crystals would be present in the joint fluid. If joint fluid tests show bacteria, it may mean that a person has *infectious (reactive) arthritis*, a form of arthritis caused by a bacterial infection.

Lyme serology test. The Lyme serology blood test looks for particular antibodies that react to *Borrelia burgdorferi,* the bacterium that causes *Lyme disease*. Lyme disease, resulting from a bite from an infected tick, can cause fever, muscle and joint pain, fatigue and other symptoms.

Rheumatoid factor test (also known as RA latex test). Blood testing may reveal the presence of the rheumatoid factor autoantibody, or RF. About 80 per cent of people with rheumatoid arthritis produce large amounts of rheumatoid factor, so this test may indicate a diagnosis of RA. However, some people who do not have RA also test positive for this autoantibody, so the test doesn't confirm the disease without other evidence.

Tissue typing test. Tissue typing is used to confirm the presence of certain genetic markers or signs in the blood that may indicate certain diseases. If the test reveals that the person has a marker called HLA-B27, for example, it may indicate a diagnosis of ankylosing spondylitis or of reactive arthritis, a disease marked by painful inflammation of the joints, and sometimes of the eyes and urethra.

Uric acid test. In this test, levels of uric acid, a waste product produced by cells in the body,

are measured. If uric acid levels are high, it may indicate the person has gout.

Urinalysis. This general testing of the urine can help to detect kidney or urinary tract infections, or other similar health problems that cause changes to your urine. High levels of certain elements, such as uric acid or protein, can aid in diagnosis of disease.

Imaging Tests

X-rays and similar tests use radiation – often in extremely small amounts – to produce images that reveal the inside of your body. Doctors use these images to examine the joints and other structures for signs of damage that may be causing pain. These tests are administered and reviewed by a specialist known as a *radiologist.* If you need to have a special imaging test, your doctor will refer you to a radiologist to perform the necessary procedure.

Below is a rundown of some of the most common imaging tests used in diagnosing chronic pain conditions, such as back problems, arthritis and related diseases.

X-rays. X-ray images, or *radiographs*, are created when controlled electromagnetic radiation is beamed through the part of the body being examined. X-rays are used to diagnose many diseases and injuries, from arthritis to a broken bone. Your doctor can use radiographs to view the bones and connective tissue that make up your joints.

An X-ray image can show problems that could be causing pain. X-rays can indicate the presence of a *tumour* (which could be cancerous or *malignant,* or non-cancerous or *benign*), or mass, that may be causing pain by pressing against organs, bones or tissues. X-rays can also show fractures (or breaks) in bones. A fracture in a vertebra, one of the bones that make up the spine, might cause back pain. X-rays are limited somewhat in their ability to reveal some soft-tissue problems, but they can assess some soft-tissue masses pressing against bones, as well as calcification (or hardening) within soft tissues that may be causing pain. In some cases, other, more precise new imaging methods may help the doctor more.

X-rays can reveal various problems associated with a chronic disease such as osteoarthritis. By reviewing the type of joint damage seen on your X-ray, doctors can pinpoint the disease that is causing your pain. By looking at an X-ray of a joint affected by osteoarthritis, a doctor can see if the space between the two bones that make up the joint is too narrow and uneven due to the wear and damage OA causes to the cartilage in the joint. X-rays might also reveal bone spurs – painful outcroppings at the ends of bones. X-ray images showing inflammation in the joints of the spine might suggest ankylosing spondylitis or a similar disease.

Whilst X-rays are very commonly used in diagnosis, X-ray technology does involve exposure to radiation. Read the section 'Are X-rays Harmful?' on page 39 to learn more about the risks and what precautions you should take.

DEXA (dual energy X-ray absorptiometry). DEXA scans are a very reliable way to diagnose osteoporosis, a disease marked by thinning bones. For this reason, many people refer to DEXA scans as 'bone density tests'. People with osteoporosis are at an increased risk for serious bone breaks, and DEXA scans help to assess that risk. The images measure bone density to determine if your bones are becoming weaker because the 'honeycomb' of the inside of the bones has become fragile.

Women who may be at risk for osteoporosis – those at or past the menopause or those who have taken bone-thinning corticosteroid medications for diseases such as rheumatoid arthritis – are most likely to have DEXA scans to diagnose the disease.

DEXA scans use less radiation than a traditional X-ray. When you have a DEXA scan, you lie on a table while the DEXA imaging machine passes over you. It is not painful and lasts only about 15 to 20 minutes.

MRI. You've probably seen the term MRI (short for magnetic resonance imaging) often in the news, especially on the sports pages. It is the preferred type of imaging in sports players, as it is virtually risk-free because it doesn't use radiation. These scans help see a much more detailed internal image of the body than plain X-rays, so problems associated with soft tissues as well as with bones can be diagnosed.

When you have an MRI scan, you lie on a long, narrow table. The table moves you into a big, enclosed tube where a strong magnet passes a force through your body. The mag-

ARE X-RAYS HARMFUL?

Because X-rays beam radiation through part of your body in order to create the image that your doctor reviews, it is understandable that you would be concerned about the risk. Too much exposure to radiation could harm the body, even leading to diseases such as cancer. Most people will not have nearly enough X-rays to incur this risk.

Even so, doctors should use X-rays only when necessary, and take only enough X-rays to get the job done without putting you at too much risk for radiation's possi-ble effects. The radiographer will 'shoot' only the area of your body that needs examination. In some cases, they will cover parts of your torso and lower body (especially where your sex organs sit) with a lead apron to shield you from excess radiation that could be harmful.

If you are a woman, it's important that you tell the radiographer if you think you may be pregnant. Radiation from an X-ray could be harmful to a fetus. So speak up if you are pregnant or even if you think you might be pregnant.

netic force creates a computer image of a cross-section of the area of your body your doctor needs to examine. The image is very detailed. The whole process may take up to an hour. Because of the length of the process, some people find MRI uncomfortable, particularly those who are claustrophobic or fearful of enclosed spaces. A new MRI machine called 'open MRI' is less confining. Open MRI may not produce images of the same detail as traditional MRI, however, and it is not available in some areas.

Many people with arthritis or related diseases have MRI scans to determine different pain-causing problems. Bone loss, knee injuries and other types of joint problems can be diagnosed through MRI technology.

MRI does not use radiation, so in some ways it is safer than X-rays. However, there are other potential problems with using MRI. If you have a pacemaker or other type of metal implant (such as those used in joint replacements or spine surgery) within your body, you may not be able to have MRI because of the magnetic element. Your doctor or the MRI operators should ask you if you have either of these devices, but speak up if they do not ask.

CT or CAT Scan. Computed axial tomography, commonly called CT or CAT scans, may be used in some cases to diagnose painful conditions or injuries to bones or internal organs. CT scans are similar to X-rays, but use a computer to create a more detailed image of the internal structures of the body or a specific area. CT scans may be useful in diagnosing back or spine problems such as fractured vertebrae, or to identify tumours. CT scans and MRI can be more expensive than other types of scans, so they are often reserved for investigating problems that cannot be diagnosed using regular X-rays.

Bone scans, myelography and discography. Bone scans, myelograms and discograms are imaging techniques that involve injecting a special dye into the body to illuminate or highlight areas of inflammation or damage. These techniques are often used in diagnosing painful back or spinal cord problems. They may be used prior to surgery to help the doctor pinpoint the precise location of the injury or problem.

Bone scans involve injecting a small amount of radioactive dye into a vein in your arm. The doctor allows the dye to circulate through your body for a couple of hours. The radioactive dye will collect in the bones. Then, he will use a scanner, a camera-like instrument, to view the painful area. The scanner produces a picture either on a computer screen or on film. The scan helps the doctor see any area of bone that has an increase in blood flow and bone-forming cell activity. These changes could indicate a tumour, infection or vertebral fracture.

Discography shows problems with the spinal discs, a common source of serious chronic pain. In a discogram, the radiologist injects into the disc or discs being examined a

dye that shows up as opaque on an imaging scan. The doctor then obtains a CT scan. The dye should illuminate any tears, scars or changes in the disc that may be causing pain.

In *myelography*, the doctor injects a special radiopaque dye into the spinal canal. This dye looks opaque on a standard X-ray, while the bones and tissues around it appear translucent. The dye can highlight a painful condition such as a herniated disc or nerve root compression.

Unlike other imaging tests, these three tests are invasive. Like surgery, this term means that the doctor must enter the body to perform the tests. Invasive tests have some potential for complications, such as infection. Your doctor should discuss the potential for these risks with you beforehand.

Microfocal radiography and thermography. Some newer imaging tests allow doctors to detect damage such as deteriorated cartilage, joint erosions, inflamed soft tissues or synovitis (inflamed joint lining) at early stages, before these problems would show up on X-rays.

Microfocal radiography uses enhanced resolution scanning and a finer grain of film to produce a sharper image of the painful area. However, microfocal radiography equipment may not be found outside specialist centres.

Thermography uses infrared technology to detect the heat that can be associated with painful inflammation. The scan can detect increased heat loss from the skin surface in a painful area, indicating inflammation. Neuropathic pain can sometimes cause a 'cold spot' to appear on the scan.

Ultrasonography. A much less invasive scanning technique is ultrasonography or ultrasound, which uses high-frequency sound waves to produce pictures (called *sonograms*) of joints, muscles, organs and other parts of the body. The echo of the sound waves off the tissues produces the visual picture. These waves are harmless to the body. Ultrasonography is commonly used to view a fetus during pregnancy.

Doctors can use ultrasonography to diagnose a number of problems that may be causing pain, including ligament tears, subtle joint damage and more. Ultrasonography allows doctors to see inside the body without any invasive techniques, such as needles, dyes or exposure to radiation.

Tests Involving Minor Surgery

The following tests involve having a small operation. Don't be alarmed: these tests involve only small cuts and usually can be done in a short time that won't require you to be admitted to hospital. Your recovery should be quick and any additional pain from the test should be very minor.

Arthroscopy. On the sports page where you read about your favourite striker having an MRI scan to diagnose his knee injury, you may also have read about him having arthroscopy or arthroscopic surgery. This is a very common, minimally invasive procedure that helps doctors diagnose or correct problems that cause serious pain in joints such as knees, hips, elbows and shoulders.

Your doctor may refer you to an orthopaedic surgeon (a doctor who specializes in performing operations on bones and joints) for arthroscopy or other types of surgery. The surgeon will make a small incision and insert a thin tube with a light at the end, called an *arthroscope*, directly into your painful joint. You may be awake during this procedure, but the area will be numbed so you won't feel anything. People undergoing arthroscopy usually don't have to stay overnight in the hospital; they just have the procedure as an outpatient, staying for a few hours. Recovery from the surgery takes only a day or so.

The arthroscope is like a little camera, and it sends an image to a TV screen in the operating room. Your surgeon sees what's going on inside your joint on the screen, and is able to move the tiny arthroscope around as needed. The surgeon may also insert other instruments to cut away ragged cartilage or to mend torn tissue.

Biopsy. A biopsy is when a doctor removes a small piece of tissue to examine it for clues to the diagnosis. Biopsies involve surgery, but it's usually quick and the incisions (cuts made during surgery) are often small.

Your doctor may need to perform a biopsy to diagnose diseases affecting joints, muscles, skin or blood vessels. In addition, doctors use biopsies to remove growths to see if they are cancerous. A cyst or tumour (even if it is benign) may be the cause of severe pain in many parts of the body.

What If a Diagnosis Isn't Clear?

There are many problems that may cause your pain. Doctors have a great deal of knowledge and resources at hand to help them figure out what is wrong with their patients, but they are only human. It may take some time before you and your doctor determine what is causing your pain.

Some of the reasons why your doctor may need some time to nail down your diagnosis include:

- Different diseases have similar or even identical symptoms. Your doctor may need to perform a number of different tests to figure out which disease you have.

- One person's disease may not be the same as another's. You may have a herniated disc in your spine that is causing you occasional pain that sends you reaching for a cooling gel to apply to it. Your neighbour may also have a herniated disc, but experiences so much pain that he needs to go to bed for three days every time it flares up. You both have the same problem but may not experience the same level of pain or exactly the same symptoms.

- Diseases and injuries don't keep to a schedule. You may have osteoarthritis that has developed much faster than is typical, causing unexpected joint damage and a lot of pain. Your doctor may not be used to seeing patients with osteoarthritis who have

your level of pain or movement problems. So your doctor may need to review all the symptoms carefully to determine your exact problem and its extent.

Your pain may continue while you undergo tests and search for the cause. Speak openly with your doctor about your concerns. Ask if there is something you can take to ease your pain while he performs tests and rules out the wrong causes.

There are many mild, pain-relieving drugs that can ease your discomfort with few, if any, side effects. The most common is paracetamol. Ask your doctor if it's OK for you to take paracetamol now for your pain and if he has any guidelines for you for taking this drug. It's available over the counter, so you don't need a prescription. Use caution, however; heavy paracetamol use may be dangerous and lead to liver disease. Talk to your doctor about your options until a diagnosis can be determined and a course of treatment started. We'll learn more about this and other useful drugs for treating your pain in the next chapter.

Expert Patients Programme

The Expert Patients Programme (EPP) is an NHS-based scheme that was set up in 2002. Based on research in the UK and the USA that found that people with chronic illness are often best equipped to know what they need in managing their own condition, the Expert Patients Programme provides them with the skills to manage their illnesses on a day-to-day basis.

In this scheme, patients and doctors and other health-care professionals work together in partnership to develop ways to help people manage their condition in the best possible way according to each person's own needs.

Expert patient courses to learn how to become an 'expert patient' take place in 2½-hour sessions once a week for six weeks. They are led by people who, themselves, live with a chronic health condition. To find out more about the scheme and to discover whether there is a scheme in your area, contact the Programme (details in the Resources section at the back of the book).

Developing Your Pain-Management Plan

Once your doctor has performed the necessary tests and discussed your pain and other symptoms, hopefully he will have made a diagnosis. When you have a diagnosis, you have a name for the cause of your pain, and that's very important. You may have lived with serious pain for a long time without knowing why. You couldn't tell others, including your spouse, children, employer and friends, why you hurt. So other people may not have understood the intensity and nature of your pain. They might have thought you were exaggerating or complaining unnecessarily, which can be frustrating.

That's why getting the right diagnosis is important. You don't want just to treat the pain – you want to manage your pain while treating its cause. But once you have a diagnosis, you move on to Step Three, creating your pain-management plan. (Sometimes it isn't possible to pinpoint the cause but you can still develop a pain-management plan.)

What is a pain-management plan? It's not just a course of drugs; it's a comprehensive strategy for controlling your chronic pain on a day-to-day basis. Managing pain will require a long-term commitment from you. You will need to take your medications as prescribed. You will need to keep your body as healthy and fit as possible. You will need to get enough rest and keep your stress in check.

It's possible that your pain will never completely go away. But you can find treatments and strategies – not just drugs – that may make your condition manageable for you. You will find that some treatments and techniques work to control your pain and some do not. The strategies that work will go into your pain-management plan. Discard the techniques that don't work, but do so only in conjunction with your doctor.

Your pain-management plan can be something you keep in your head, or you can write it down and keep a document of everything you do. We suggest that you do keep a written record of your pain-management plan. Keeping track of the drugs or supplements you take, the complementary therapies (such as acupuncture, TENS or chiropractic) you use, and the exercises you do will help you and your doctor get a clearer picture of what is working for you. Think of this document as a journal of your pain and your efforts to control that pain. Keep track of what you do and when you do it. Note the effects. Does the prescription drug your doctor gave you work to relieve your pain? Do you feel pain after your exercise routine? What kind of pain? How long does it last? Every detail will help you note patterns in your pain and identify techniques that work.

Your pain-management plan should have several components. It can include drug therapy, including prescription drugs from your doctor or over-the-counter drugs purchased at the pharmacists. (We explain some of the differences between these types of drugs in the next chapter.) Your plan should include guidance from your doctor about when you should you take what drug and how much you should take.

Your plan should include more than just medications. Although you might like to take a pill for your pain and forget about it, most doctors would not recommend that approach. Many analgesic drugs have side effects, and they may not control your pain adequately by themselves.

To be successful, a pain-management plan should be comprehensive. Pain may be caused by a physical problem, but your overall health and lifestyle habits can greatly affect your level of pain. Pain can get worse if you smoke, don't exercise or are overweight. Changing these factors can help you control your pain.

Physiotherapy and *occupational therapy* are important options to explore as you and your doctor devise your pain-management plan. A physiotherapist can create a customized exercise plan to improve your physical health or help reduce pain. An occupational therapist can work with you to adjust the way you do your everyday activities to make them easier (for example, making cutlery handles larger so that you can grip them more easily) and to reduce risk of injury and lessen pain. Either type of therapist may be able to fit you with customized *splints* or *braces* to place around wrists, knees, back or ankles to offer support and stability and help you manage pain.

There are many so-called natural or complementary therapies that you might try. These include herbal supplements – natural ingredients designed to help control pain, reduce inflammation or help you relax. (These remedies, while considered 'natural,' still carry risks. Chapter 7 discusses this subject in depth.) Other complementary therapies for pain include *acupuncture*, an ancient Chinese pain-control method involving the insertion of fine needles into your skin, and *chiropractic,* a more contemporary method of adjusting the spine to relieve pain and pressure; they are discussed in Chapter 8.

Exercise can help build up your muscles so they can support weakened or damaged joints, and exercise can increase your flexibility so that tendons, ligaments and muscles can function more effectively, with less risk of painful injury. Your doctor, in addition to a physiotherapist, can offer you specific exercises to perform to ease your pain.

Pain is often worsened, or sometimes even caused, by stress and tension. Therefore, methods to reduce your tension can help control your pain. All of these important components of your pain-management plan –

exercise, diet, healthy habits, relaxation therapies – don't involve drugs or chemicals of any kind. So these therapies can be a natural boost to your pain-control efforts.

Pain Management Programme

The Pain Management Programme run by the British Pain Society is a rehabilitation programme for people with chronic pain that has not been resolved by other treatments. Its aim is to reduce the disability and distress caused by long-term pain by teaching people physical, psychological and practical techniques to help them improve their quality of life. Although pain relief isn't the primary goal of this programme, it has been demonstrated in those who have participated in the programme.

The programme, delivered by a multi-disciplinary team of experienced health-care professionals, runs for twelve mornings over a period of eight weeks.

For more information, contact the British Pain Society (details in the Resources section). If you would like to attend a programme, ask your doctor for a referral.

Whilst your pain-management plan should be comprehensive, drugs are an important component of controlling chronic pain. The next two chapters explore the many drugs available to treat chronic pain and its sources. We also discuss issues associated with drug treatment. These issues include how to use your medicine properly and how to differentiate between the various treatments available to find the best one for you.

SAMPLE PAIN QUESTIONNAIRE

(Reprinted, with minor amendments, with permission of The Cleveland Clinic Foundation, Department of Pain Management)

The following questionnaire is an example of the type of extensive, comprehensive pain survey your doctor might give you as you begin the diagnosis and treatment process.

Outcomes Questionnaire: 1 3 6 month

Patient Name: _____ **Date:** _____

1. Where is your pain located? Tick all that apply:

❏ Head	❏ Hand	❏ Pelvis
❏ Face	❏ Chest	❏ Buttock
❏ Neck	❏ Upper back	❏ Genitalia
❏ Shoulder	❏ Abdomen	❏ Leg
❏ Arm	❏ Lower back	❏ Foot

2. In general, would you say your health is:

❏ Excellent
❏ Very good
❏ Good
❏ Fair
❏ Poor

3. Compared to one year ago, how would you rate your health in general now?

❏ Much better now than one year ago
❏ Somewhat better now than one year ago
❏ About the same now as one year ago
❏ Somewhat worse now than one year ago
❏ Much worse now than one year ago

The following items are about activities you might do in a typical day. Does your health now limit you in these activities? If so, how much?

4. Vigorous activities, such as running, lifting heavy objects, participating in strenuous sports:

❑ Yes, limited a lot
❑ Yes, limited a little
❑ No, not limited at all

5. Moderate activities, such as moving a table, pushing a vacuum cleaner, bowling or playing golf:

❑ Yes, limited a lot
❑ Yes, limited a little
❑ No, not limited at all

6. Lifting or carrying groceries:

❑ Yes, limited a lot
❑ Yes, limited a little
❑ No, not limited at all

7. Climbing several flights of stairs:

❑ Yes, limited a lot
❑ Yes, limited a little
❑ No, not limited at all

8. Climbing one flight of stairs:

❑ Yes, limited a lot
❑ Yes, limited a little
❑ No, not limited at all

9. Bending, kneeling or stooping:

❑ Yes, limited a lot
❑ Yes, limited a little
❑ No, not limited at all

10. Walking more than a mile:

❑ Yes, limited a lot
❑ Yes, limited a little
❑ No, not limited at all

11. Walking several blocks:

❑ Yes, limited a lot
❑ Yes, limited a little
❑ No, not limited at all

12. Walking one block:

❑ Yes, limited a lot
❑ Yes, limited a little
❑ No, not limited at all

13. Bathing or dressing myself:

❑ Yes, limited a lot
❑ Yes, limited a little
❑ No, not limited at all

During the <u>past four weeks</u>, have you had any of the following problems with your work or other regular daily activities as a result of your physical health?

14. Cut down on the amount of time you spend on work or other activities:

❑ Yes
❑ No

15. Accomplished less than you would like:

❑ Yes
❑ No

16. Were limited in the kind of work or other activities:

❑ Yes
❑ No

17. Had difficulty performing the work or other activities (i.e. it took extra effort):

❏ Yes
❏ No

During the <u>past four weeks</u>, have you had any of the following problems with your work or other regular daily activities <u>as a result of any emotional problems</u> (such as feeling depressed or anxious)?

18. Cut down on the amount of time you spend on work or other activities:

❏ Yes
❏ No

19. Accomplished less than you would like:

❏ Yes
❏ No

20. Didn't do work or other activities as carefully as usual:

❏ Yes
❏ No

21. During the <u>past four weeks</u>, to what extent have your physical health or emotional problems interfered with your normal social activities with family, friends, neighbours or groups?

❏ Not at all
❏ Slightly
❏ Moderately
❏ Quite a bit
❏ Extremely

22. How much pain have you had in the <u>past four weeks</u>?

❏ None
❏ Very mild
❏ Mild
❏ Moderate
❏ Severe
❏ Very severe

23. During the <u>past four weeks</u>, how much did <u>pain</u> interfere with your normal work (including both work outside the home and housework)?

❏ Not at all
❏ Slightly
❏ Moderately
❏ Quite a bit
❏ Extremely

The following questions are about how you feel and how things have been with you during the <u>past four weeks</u>. For each question, please give the one answer that comes closest to the way you have been feeling.
How much of the time during the <u>past four weeks</u>:

24. Did you feel full of energy?

❏ All of the time
❏ Most of the time
❏ A good bit of the time
❏ Some of the time
❏ A little bit of the time
❏ None of the time

25. Have you been a very nervous person?

- ❏ All of the time
- ❏ Most of the time
- ❏ A good bit of the time
- ❏ Some of the time
- ❏ A little bit of the time
- ❏ None of the time

26. Have you felt so down in the dumps that nothing could cheer you up?

- ❏ All of the time
- ❏ Most of the time
- ❏ A good bit of the time
- ❏ Some of the time
- ❏ A little bit of the time
- ❏ None of the time

27. Have you felt calm and peaceful?

- ❏ All of the time
- ❏ Most of the time
- ❏ A good bit of the time
- ❏ Some of the time
- ❏ A little bit of the time
- ❏ None of the time

28. Did you have a lot of energy?

- ❏ All of the time
- ❏ Most of the time
- ❏ A good bit of the time
- ❏ Some of the time
- ❏ A little bit of the time
- ❏ None of the time

29. Have you felt downhearted and blue?

- ❏ All of the time
- ❏ Most of the time
- ❏ A good bit of the time
- ❏ Some of the time
- ❏ A little bit of the time
- ❏ None of the time

30. Did you feel worn out?

- ❏ All of the time
- ❏ Most of the time
- ❏ A good bit of the time
- ❏ Some of the time
- ❏ A little bit of the time
- ❏ None of the time

31. Have you been a happy person?

- ❏ All of the time
- ❏ Most of the time
- ❏ A good bit of the time
- ❏ Some of the time
- ❏ A little bit of the time
- ❏ None of the time

32. Did you feel tired?

- ❏ All of the time
- ❏ Most of the time
- ❏ A good bit of the time
- ❏ Some of the time
- ❏ A little bit of the time
- ❏ None of the time

33. During the <u>past four weeks</u>, how much of the time has your <u>physical health or emotional problems</u> interfered with your social activities (such as visiting with friends, relatives, etc.)?

- ❏ All of the time
- ❏ Most of the time
- ❏ A good bit of the time
- ❏ Some of the time
- ❏ A little bit of the time
- ❏ None of the time

How <u>true or false</u> is each of the following statements for you?

34. I seem to get ill a little easier than other people.

- ❏ Definitely true
- ❏ Mostly true
- ❏ Don't know
- ❏ Mostly false
- ❏ Definitely false

35. I am as healthy as anybody I know.

- ❏ Definitely true
- ❏ Mostly true
- ❏ Don't know
- ❏ Mostly false
- ❏ Definitely false

36. I expect my health to get worse.

- ❏ Definitely true
- ❏ Mostly true
- ❏ Don't know
- ❏ Mostly false
- ❏ Definitely false

37. My health is excellent.

- ❏ Definitely true
- ❏ Mostly true
- ❏ Don't know
- ❏ Mostly false
- ❏ Definitely false

38. What is your current work status?
Tick all that apply.

- ❏ Working full time
- ❏ Working part time
- ❏ Volunteer working
- ❏ Retired
- ❏ Vocational rehabilitation
- ❏ School
- ❏ Not working

39. Since your last clinic visit, have you required any of the following?
Tick all that apply.

- ❏ Medication adjustment
- ❏ Hospitalization
- ❏ Surgery
- ❏ Unscheduled doctor visit
- ❏ Accident and Emergency visit

40. Medication Assessment
What drugs are you using regularly (more than twice a week)?
Check YES or NO for each category.

Anticonvulsants?   ❏ YES ❏ NO
Amount and type: _____
_____

Antiarrythmics?   ❏ YES ❏ NO
Amount and type: _____
_____

Opiates? ❑ YES ❑ NO

Amount and type: _____

_____

Benzodiazepines/
tranquillizers? ❑ YES ❑ NO

Amount and type: _____

_____

Antidepressants? ❑ YES ❑ NO

Amount and type: _____

_____

Non-steroidal anti-
inflammatory drugs? ❑ YES ❑ NO

Amount and type: _____

_____

Sleeping pills? ❑ YES ❑ NO

Amount and type: _____

_____

41. Alcohol Assessment

Within the last month, have
you used alcohol? ❑ YES ❑ NO

Type of alcohol. Tick all that apply.
- ❑ Beer
- ❑ Wine
- ❑ Spirits (i.e. whisky)
- ❑ Not applicable

How many alcoholic drinks a week do you
consume?
- ❑ None
- ❑ Fewer than the recommended limit*

- ❑ About the recommended limit*
- ❑ A few more than the recommended
limit*
- ❑ Many more than the recommended
limit*

  * 14 units for women; 21 units for men

42. Support System Assessment

Do you attend self-help meetings?

- ❑ Never
- ❑ Almost never
- ❑ At least once a month
- ❑ Several times a month

43. Treatment Helpfulness Questionnaire

How would you rate the quality of the
following treatments received? One
being of the lowest quality, 10 being
of the highest quality. If not received,
leave blank.

Over all
1 2 3 4 5 6 7 8 9 10

Medical assessment and treatment
1 2 3 4 5 6 7 8 9 10

Psychology assessment
1 2 3 4 5 6 7 8 9 10

Physiotherapy assessment and treatment
1 2 3 4 5 6 7 8 9 10

Visits to doctor
1 2 3 4 5 6 7 8 9 10

Medical diagnostic tests
(i.e. thermography)
1 2 3 4 5 6 7 8 9 10

44. How satisfied are you with the information you have been given about your condition?

- ❏ Very satisfied
- ❏ Satisfied
- ❏ Relatively satisfied
- ❏ Somewhat dissatisfied
- ❏ Very dissatisfied

45. How satisfied are you with the treatment you have received for your condition?

- ❏ Very satisfied
- ❏ Satisfied
- ❏ Relatively satisfied
- ❏ Somewhat dissatisfied
- ❏ Very dissatisfied

46. How satisfied are you with the overall medical care you have received at the pain clinic?

- ❏ Very satisfied
- ❏ Satisfied
- ❏ Relatively satisfied
- ❏ Somewhat satisfied
- ❏ Very dissatisfied

47. When was the <u>first time</u> in your life that the pain problem for which you are seeking medical attention first occurred?

- ❏ Less than one month ago
- ❏ Between one and six months ago
- ❏ Between six months and a year ago
- ❏ Between one and two years ago
- ❏ Between two and three years ago
- ❏ Between three and four years ago
- ❏ Between four and five years ago
- ❏ Between five and ten years ago

- ❏ Between ten and twenty years ago
- ❏ Between twenty and thirty years ago
- ❏ More than thirty years ago

48. When did the current episode of the pain problem for which you are seeking medical attention first occur?

- ❏ Less than one month ago
- ❏ Between one and six months ago
- ❏ Between six months and a year ago
- ❏ Between one and two years ago
- ❏ Between two and three years ago
- ❏ Between three and four years ago
- ❏ Between four and five years ago
- ❏ Between five and ten years ago
- ❏ Between ten and twenty years ago
- ❏ Between twenty and thirty years ago
- ❏ More than thirty years ago

49. During the <u>past four weeks</u>, how many days have you missed work?

- ❏ None
- ❏ 1–3 days
- ❏ 4–7 days (once a week)
- ❏ 8–11 days (twice a week)
- ❏ 12–15 days (three times a week)
- ❏ 16 days or more (daily or almost daily)
- ❏ Not relevant

50. During the <u>past four weeks</u>, how many days have you had to cut down on your time at work (arrive late or leave early)?

- ❏ None
- ❏ 1–3 days
- ❏ 4–7 days (once a week)
- ❏ 8–11 days (twice a week)
- ❏ 12–15 days (three times a week)

❏ 16 days or more (daily or almost daily)

❏ Not relevant

51. During the <u>past four weeks</u>, how many days have you been unable to meet work deadlines?

❏ None

❏ 1–3 days

❏ 4–7 days (once a week)

❏ 8–11 days (twice a week)

❏ 12–15 days (three times a week)

❏ 16 days or more (daily or almost daily)

❏ Not relevant

52. During the <u>past four weeks</u>, which of the following terms describes your disability status?

❏ Not disabled

❏ Partially disabled

❏ Totally disabled

❏ Temporarily disabled

❏ Permanently disabled

53. During the <u>past four weeks</u>, which of the following terms describes your employment status?

❏ Unemployed

❏ Student

❏ Gainfully employed/full-time

❏ Gainfully employed/part-time

❏ Volunteer employment full-time

❏ Volunteer employment part-time

54. During the <u>past four weeks</u>, how many times have you received care in an A & E department?

❏ None

❏ Once

❏ Twice

❏ Three times

❏ Four times

55. During the <u>past four weeks</u>, how many times have you been admitted to hospital?

❏ None

❏ Once

❏ Twice

❏ Three times

❏ Four times

56. During the <u>past four weeks</u>, how many times have you been to see health-care providers (doctors, nurses, therapists, etc.)?

❏ None

❏ 1–3 times

❏ 4–7 times (once a week)

❏ 8–11 times (twice a week)

❏ 12–15 times (three times a week)

❏ 16–19 times (four times a week)

❏ 20 times or more (daily or almost daily)

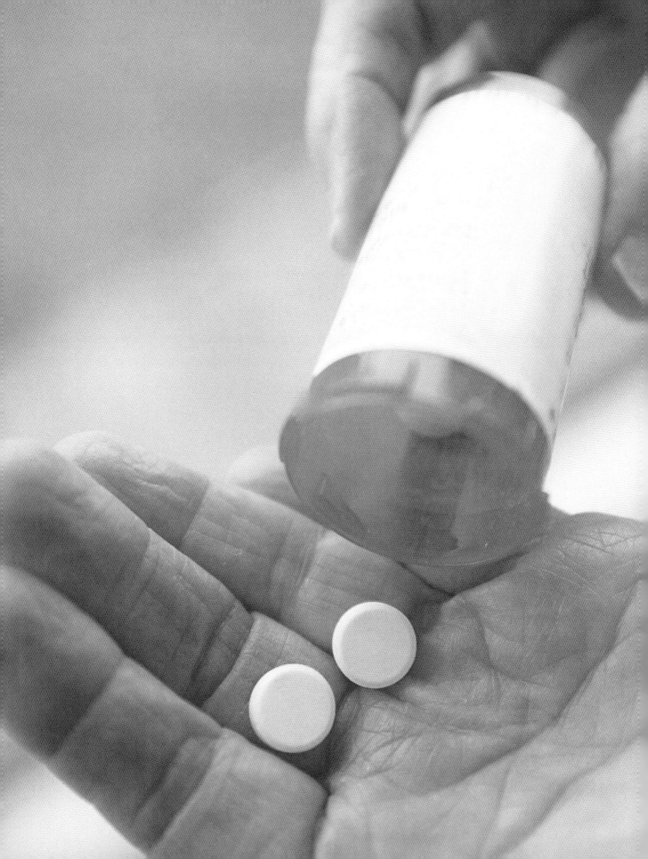

Taking Drugs For Pain

3

CHAPTER 3: TAKING DRUGS FOR PAIN

There are many ways you can treat your pain: drugs, 'natural' treatments, lifestyle changes that can reduce or help you manage pain, new medical methods for curbing pain, and surgical treatments.

Treatment with a drug – or you may call them medicines or medications – is probably the most common approach to relieve chronic pain. Most drugs come in pill form, but your doctor might give you injections of pain-treating drugs (for example, a corticosteroid for plantar fasciitis). Some drugs are available over the counter – without a prescription from your doctor. Others are available only with a prescription. If you pay for your prescriptions, it may be that you can obtain certain drugs that your doctor has prescribed more cheaply by buying them 'over the counter'. Ask your pharmacist.

Another possibility is to buy a prescription 'season ticket': you pay a fixed sum in advance, and that covers you for all NHS prescriptions for a certain period. This scheme is worth it if you have 6 or more items in four months or 15 or more items in a year. At the time of writing (2006) the cost was £6.65 per item or £34.65 for four months or £95.30 for a year. Apply for this pre-payment certificate on form FP95, available at most chemist/ pharmacist shops and main post offices or from your Primary Care Trust.

In this chapter we discuss important terms about drugs, so you will know what you are taking and what you are buying. You'll learn what drugs are available to fight your pain and treat the underlying causes of pain. The good news is that there are thousands of drugs on the market today, and your doctor has the knowledge and experience to work with you to find the right drugs to treat your problem.

WHAT IS A DRUG?

Drugs are chemicals or substances that affect the structure or functioning of your body. The drugs we are talking about in this chapter are *therapeutic drugs,* or drugs designed to treat problems or relieve pain. Doctors developed the first drugs from natural sources, such as trees, flowers or minerals. In recent history, scientists began developing more sophisticated drugs to target specific functions in the body in an effort to treat problems. Some drugs are *synthetic*, or man-made, versions of natural substances, even substances found within your own body, such as hormones.

Although there may be many drugs available to treat a problem or condition – for instance to reduce painful inflammation – you may find that one medication is more effective for you than others. Why? Even though some drugs do the same thing, they may treat the problem in a different way or have a different active ingredient. To add to the confusion, some medicines are exactly the same except for their brand name (see p. 59).

Your doctor can help you sort through the confusion to find the best medication to treat your pain.

As we discuss drugs, we will list the generic or scientific name of the drug first, and then list the brand names of the drug in italics and in parentheses. Many drugs come in numerous brands. Generic, or non-name-brand, versions of many drugs are available. In most cases, there may be no difference except the price.

Drugs: Important Things To Know

Simply put, a drug is any medicine you take to help your pain or other problems. Whilst you may hear the word 'drug' used in discussions about marijuana, cocaine or other 'street drugs', we're talking about helpful drugs that can treat your pain. Because pain medications can be serious and powerful, it's important for you and your doctor to work together to choose the right medicines for you.

Drugs can come in many forms: pills, injections, liquid drinks, creams or other formulations. As we learned in Chapter 1, some drugs can help to narrow or close the 'pain gate' that allows pain signals to pass into the brain. These drugs actually decrease the degree to which you feel pain. They 'dull' the pain. Other drugs may work to modify the internal problems that are causing pain in the first place – such as inflammation, joint damage or infections.

In the last ten years or so, the number of drugs available to treat health problems has grown tremendously. There are thousands of drugs on the market and more on the way. Your doctor knows the right ones for you to choose from. As you and your doctor work together to find the right treatments for your pain, you may have some questions about how to take the drugs your doctor prescribes, what the drugs do and what effects they may have on your body. Be sure to speak up when you have questions about your drugs. It's important to take your drugs just as your doctor prescribes, and to know what side effects or cautions to be aware of. Ask your doctor to explain everything about your drugs during your appointment.

Drugs, whether ones that your doctor prescribes or ones that you buy without a prescription, should be only one part of that overall pain-management plan, albeit a very important part. A comprehensive pain-management plan includes not just drugs, but also regular exercise, a proper diet, stress control methods, and more.

Below are some important matters to consider as you and your doctor explore medicines to treat your pain or the conditions that cause your pain.

Prescription vs over-the-counter drugs. An over-the-counter drug is a drug that does not require a prescription. These medicines include common drugs such as aspirin, ibuprofen or paracetamol, medicines for stomach upset or creams for muscle pain. They are available at your supermarket and local shop as well as the pharmacists. Many of these medicines can be very helpful for relieving mild, everyday pain.

When you receive a prescription drug, you will also receive specific printed information about how to take the drug safely and effectively, and what side effects to watch for. You can ask your doctor or your pharmacist any questions you may have about the use of your drug. Over-the-counter medications also contain information about the drug, its side effects and cautions about using it. But it's up to you to read this information and ask the pharmacist questions about how to use any drug safely.

If you find that you are taking over-the-counter medicines for pain on a daily basis, or often need to take the maximum, daily, recommended dosage for relief, talk to your doctor. He may wish to prescribe a medication that is stronger and more effective. In addition, there may be other lifestyle changes you should make to help control your pain.

Just because you can buy over-the-counter drugs at the corner shop without a prescription does not mean they are not powerful. If you take over-the-counter drugs for your pain, tell your doctor when you have your appointment. If you are taking prescription drugs, herbal supplements and over-the-counter drugs for the same pain, you may be taking too much of the same active ingredient. That's why it's important to tell your doctor about everything you take for pain.

Ask the pharmacist. This licensed professional fills the prescriptions from your doctor at pharmacies. A pharmacist has years of specialized education and is the only person licensed to dispense prescription drugs. Pharmacies often have assistants who can answer certain questions about your drugs. However, if you pick up your medicine at the pharmacy and have questions about how to take the drug or what side effects it may have, you should ask to speak to the pharmacist. Although pharmacists often seem busy and other customers may be waiting, it's important that you fully understand how to take your drug. Ask your pharmacist any question you have about your medicine. (See also the section on p. 60.)

Active ingredients vs inactive ingredients. The *active ingredient* in a drug is the chemical or substance that treats your problem. There may be more than one active ingredient in your medication. Some medicines are combinations of various drugs designed to treat more than one symptom, or one ingredient may ward off side effects (see p. 62) of the other ingredient.

In addition to the active ingredient or ingredients in the medicine, there are inactive ingredients, also known as fillers. These inactive ingredients should be clearly listed on the drug's packaging; if you don't see them, ask your pharmacist. These ingredients may make up the rest of the pill or liquid and make it edible or tasty, may provide a protective coating to keep the medicine from irritating your tongue or stomach, or may just act as a binder to keep the pill together.

Inactive ingredients shouldn't affect you. However, if you have allergies to certain foods or shouldn't eat certain foods, such as dairy or sugar, you may wish to find out if the drugs you take contain these foods in their inactive ingredients. The drug might bother you or cause a reaction. This is rare, but it could occur.

Brand-name vs generic drugs. Many companies can sell the same drug under different names, in bottles with different labels. Essentially it's the same thing. But the price can be very different. Think of a can of peas at the supermarket. Several companies sell cans of peas. There are even generic or 'store-brand' peas. Are the peas different? Probably not. But the generic peas can be cheaper.

For some drugs, the generic form is much cheaper than the brand-name version. Is it the same drug? The active ingredient – the chemical that does the intended job in your body – should be exactly the same. However, some other ingredients in the medicine, such as fillers or dyes, may be different. (See 'Active ingredients', p. 58.)

Some prescription drugs come in both brand-name and generic forms; others only in brand-name forms. Why? When companies develop a new drug, they have to invest their money in years of research and testing to create it. They recoup this money during the first 20 years after patenting the drug, when they have an exclusive right to sell it. When this exclusivity runs out, other companies are allowed to create their own versions of the same drug. If another company has not had to spend a lot of money to research and test the drug, it can create a form of the drug at lower cost and still make a profit. That's why generic drugs are cheaper.

If your GP prescribes a brand-name (proprietary) drug by name, the pharmacist must dispense that particular preparation. If, however, the GP writes a generic name on the prescription form, the pharmacist can dispense any version of that drug. That is why you sometimes get a different-looking pill in a different box each time you get a prescription filled for the same drug.

As with prescription drugs, there are also brand-name and generic versions of many over-the-counter drugs, like paracetamol, aspirin and ibuprofen. You might see 'own-store brands' of these medicines at your local pharmacy. They can be much cheaper in price. But if you like a brand-name over-the-counter drug, you may not wish to switch to an unfamiliar product to save some money. It's up to you. Ask the pharmacist to help you compare brands if you're unsure. One way to compare these products is to review the active ingredients listed on the packaging. If the two products contain the same amount of the same medicine, they are essentially the same drug.

Repeat prescriptions. Your GP's surgery will have a system for ordering repeat prescriptions. Ask at the surgery for details.

Not all items will be available this way, and for these you will have to make an appointment with your doctor. Why? Your doctor

QUICK TERMS ABOUT DRUGS

Caplet: Another word for pill, except that caplets usually have a light, edible coating that makes them easier to swallow than normal pills. They are usually oblong rather than round

Capsule: Small tube that holds precise amounts of medicine. The casing of the tube is edible and dissolves in your stomach with water or liquid. The capsule allows you to swallow exactly the right amount of medicine without tasting it (some medicines can taste pretty bad) or having it dissolve in your mouth.

Implant: A tiny device placed inside the body or under the skin that releases small amounts of medicine at regular intervals. Implants allow you to have medicine at regular intervals without having to take a pill.

Injection: A syringe or tube containing liquid medicine with a needle on the end that goes into your body. In the uncommon event that you have an injection of analgesic, it will usually be given by a nurse.

Intravenous: When medicine is inserted into the body through a needle into a vein.

Ointment, cream, gel: Terms for topical agents. An ointment can be greasy. They are rubbed on the skin.

Patches: Some pain-killing drugs are available as adhesive patches, which deliver steady doses of the drug over a period of up to seven days.

Pill: Small, compressed ball of powdered medicine that can be swallowed with liquid or, in some cases, chewed and swallowed without liquid. Pills can be coated or uncoated. Coating may be used to keep pills from dissolving in your mouth, making them easier to swallow or keeping you from tasting the inside, which may taste unpleasant. Coating may also serve to protect the

may wish you to use some medicines only for a short time. Once you have used a certain amount, if you don't find pain relief, your doctor may want to try something else. Medicines, as we learned earlier, can have side effects, so your doctor may not want you to take dose after dose of some drugs.

Some medicines carry the possibility of dependence – the person feels a physical need for the medication; or tolerance – the body lining of your stomach from the dissolving medicine.

Powder: Some over-the-counter, pain-relieving medicines come in powder form. The powder is pre-measured and contained in small packets. You dissolve the powder in water and drink the medicine as a liquid. Powdered medicine may be harder to find, but if you have trouble swallowing medicine in pill form, it may be useful.

Spray: Liquid medicine that comes out of a pump or aerosol (like a hairspray can) container. Spray medicines may be squirted up your nose, in your mouth or on your skin.

Suppository: A soft, dissolving capsule or pill meant to be inserted into the rectum. Usually, an applicator, or device to get the capsule into the rectum, is provided. Suppositories can release medicine into the bloodstream more quickly than drugs taken by mouth. They can, in some cases,

also prevent or lessen stomach upset as a side effect.

Suspension: A liquid medicine that has the active ingredient suspended or contained in an edible liquid. You swallow a prescribed amount of the suspension using a measuring spoon, the bottle's cap or a small plastic cup provided with the bottle. Suspensions may be used for small children or for adults who have trouble swallowing pills. Not all medicines are readily available in liquid form, so speak to your doctor if you struggle to swallow pills and need a liquid medicine.

Topical agent: Also known as creams, ointments, salves or rubs. Smooth, paste-like medicine that you rub on. Topical agents contain all kinds of medicine, including antibiotics, analgesics and antihistamines. They should be used topically, i.e. rubbed on the skin. They are not meant to be swallowed or inserted into the body unless the prescription says so clearly.

needs progressively higher doses to achieve the desired result. With such drugs, the doctor will want to monitor closely the patient's response, to spot quickly such an occurrence. You should discuss the benefits and possible

risks of continuing to use each drug. Your doctor may give you another prescription either for the same drug or for another medicine. Or he may suggest other methods for you to relieve pain without using more of this drug.

Side effects and cautions. All drugs or medicines can have side effects. This means you might have an unusual or unpleasant experience when you take the drug. These side effects can be anything from a rash to an upset stomach to unusual sleepiness or feeling 'hyper'. Even common, over-the-counter medicines may have side effects that are very noticeable.

Sometimes, side effects are minor. If you want pain relief, you may find the occasional side effect an acceptable trade-off. However, some side effects are very unpleasant or even dangerous to your health. These side effects may have to do with the particular drug or the necessary *dosage* required for adequate pain relief with it. Some people experience side effects that are as serious as the problem the drug was meant to treat. In those cases, alternatives must be found. To avoid this danger, researchers constantly work to develop new drugs that treat pain with less risk of dangerous side effects.

When your doctor prescribes a drug, he should talk to you about possible side effects. Ask him what you might expect. And ask what side effects should signal caution. In other words, if you experience certain side effects, you may wish to contact him immediately. Do not, though, stop taking the drug until you have spoken to your doctor. It can be dangerous to stop certain drugs suddenly.

Cautions associated with drugs – which should be clearly marked on the packaging of both over-the-counter and prescription medicines – are strong warnings not to take the drug in certain circumstances. You might also see specific warnings on the drug's packaging. These warnings state clearly what you should not do while taking this drug, such as driving, operating machinery or drinking alcohol. In addition, you will find a patient information leaflet enclosed with each prescription drug. If you need help understanding these warnings or the printed materials provided with any drug (these materials can be written in somewhat technical or medical language), ask your pharmacist.

Some drugs should not be used if you are taking certain other drugs, as the two medicines could cause a dangerous reaction when combined; for example, one drug might increase or decrease the effect of another. People with certain health conditions should only use some drugs with caution, as their health condition might worsen by taking this drug even if it is for another, unrelated health problem. For example, if you have high blood pressure and get a cold, taking certain decongestants might be problematic. The drugs you are taking for your cold might interact with medicines you take to control your high blood pressure. Or, if you take other drugs, such as tranquillizers, it might be dangerous to take the decongestant for your cold as well. These facts would be noted as cautions or precautions when considering taking the decongestant.

Questions About Your Health

Your health is important. When you're in pain, you deserve attention for that pain and, if possible, fast, effective relief. To get relief, your doctor may suggest and prescribe drugs for you to take. In order for them to be both safe and effective, it's very important that you take them as directed.

Drugs often need to be taken in a certain way in order to be effective and not cause problems in your body. For example, some drugs might cause stomach upset if you don't take them with food. Other drugs should be taken at certain intervals – such as every four to six hours – in order to work best.

All of these facts are very important. You could harm yourself if you take a drug improperly. At the very least, the drug may not work as well as it should if you don't take it as prescribed.

Your prescription will come with instructions about how to take the drug properly. This will be part of the patient information leaflet. Drug companies try to explain everything clearly, and some are working with the Plain English Society to make the leaflets easy to understand. The prescription bottle also may have instructions printed on it. If you don't fully understand the instructions, you should ask for clarification.

Do not feel badly if you don't understand what your doctor or pharmacist tells you at first about medicines or any other methods you use to relieve pain. Your doctor may not realize that you don't understand what to do unless you say so. If you don't feel comfortable talking to your doctor about the drug, ask the practice nurse or ask your pharmacist. Sometimes, when you collect your prescription, the pharmacy staff will say, 'Do you have any questions for the pharmacist?' Ask your questions then and there! The pharmacist is busy, but not too busy to do his or her job and answer your questions. Your doctor, nurses and pharmacist want you to take your medicines the right way so that you find relief and don't experience unnecessary side effects.

So don't be shy. Ask your doctor to explain what the medicine does and how to take it properly. Ask your pharmacist to explain it again when you pick up the prescription. Tell your doctor about other drugs or treatments you use for various problems. When you talk openly with your doctor, he is better informed about your health, and you are better informed about how to improve your health.

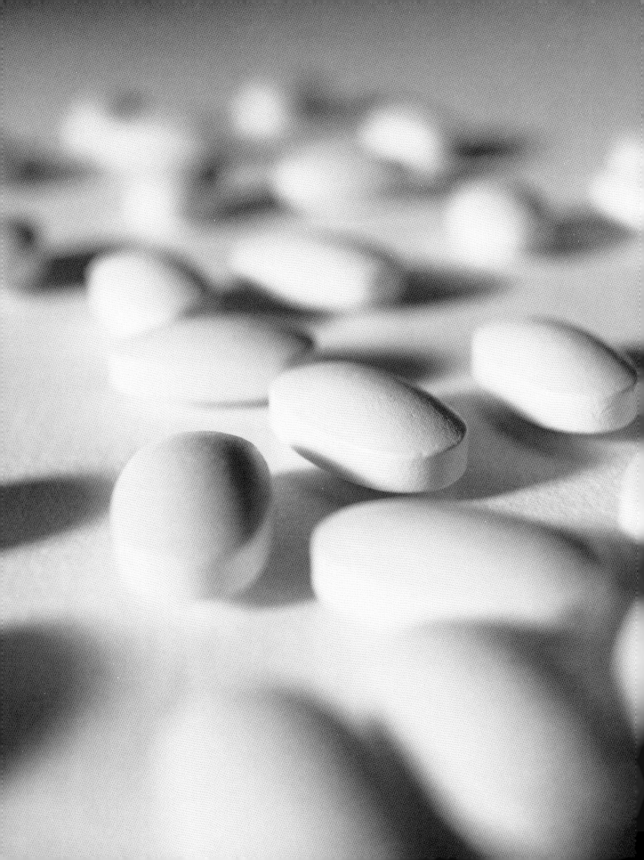

Analgesics and NSAIDs

4

CHAPTER 4: ANALGESICS AND NSAIDs

Now you know many of the different words associated with drugs. Having this vocabulary should help you better understand your conversations with your doctor and your pharmacist. It's very important that you know what drugs you are taking, and what different drugs do to help you.

In this chapter, you'll learn more about the many drugs your doctor might prescribe for pain. We also discuss some of the most common over-the-counter drugs you may be using for your pain. You will learn how these drugs work to ease your pain or to treat the underlying cause of your pain. We also discuss side effects and other cautions associated with using these drugs.

It's important for you to be involved and aware as you begin using a drug. Your responsibility doesn't end when you swallow the pill or when the sting of the injection fades. You must take your drugs according to your doctor's instructions. You should stay aware of how effectively the drug works, and take note of any side effects you experience.

In this chapter, we look at two of the most common classes of drugs used to relieve pain: analgesics and non-steroidal anti-inflammatory drugs, or NSAIDs. Chances are high that you have used one of these drugs or are using one now for pain relief. Some widely used analgesics and NSAIDs are available over the counter at a low cost, but other drugs in this class are stronger and require a prescription.

In recent years, researchers have developed new drugs in these categories that relieve pain effectively but have less risk of adverse side effects. Although they work in very different ways, medications in both categories can relieve most of the common causes of chronic pain.

ANALGESICS

If you've ever used over-the-counter pain relievers, you may have noticed the term 'analgesic' on the bottle. Analgesic simply means 'pain-fighting'. This is a group of drugs that reduce pain. They're used for many common ailments, from headaches to short-term illnesses such as colds.

As outlined in the World Health Organization's 'analgesic ladder', the objective of treatment in all types of pain is to achieve symptom control and improve the patient's quality of life. If the drugs recommended for treatment of mild pain do not treat your pain adequately, your doctor will prescribe stronger analgesics in a step-wise fashion until pain control is achieved.

Analgesic drugs may not treat the underlying cause of pain, such as reducing inflammation or treating infections. They simply work to reduce your sensation of pain. Some analgesic drugs, such as paracetamol, well known by brand names such as *Panadol,* also have *antipyretic* effects, or reducing fever or body temperature. Analgesic drugs are a very effective and important way to control chronic pain.

Aspirin

Aspirin is a salicylate, meaning that it contains salicylic acid – which comes from willow bark. It is a drug with several different properties: an analgesic, an antipyretic (it reduces fever) and also an anti-inflammatory. It is often used in adults (not advised for children under 12) for musculoskeletal pain. Aspirin may cause stomach irritation, in which case specially coated tablets may be tolerated better.

Aspirin is the most common salicylate, and aspirin was originally made from willow bark. If you have allergic reactions to aspirin, you should not take other salicylates or even herbal supplements derived from willow bark.

Children may be at risk for a dangerous disease called *Reye's syndrome* if they take aspirin. Children who are experiencing pain should be given only medicines designed for children their age (which do not contain aspirin), or given the recommended dosage of standard drugs for children their age or weight.

Paracetamol

When a medicine bottle says 'aspirin-free pain reliever,' paracetamol is the drug you are probably taking. Paracetamol is the first drug you should take for minor osteoarthritis pain. The daily dose should not exceed 4 grams of medicine. Higher doses of this drug could lead to liver disease.

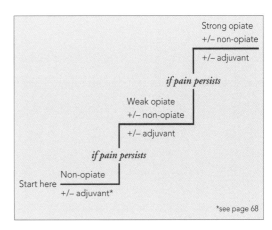

THE WORLD HEALTH ORGANIZATION
THREE-STEP ANALGESIC LADDER

Paracetamol can reduce mild to moderate pain and reduce fever, but it does not treat swelling, redness or stiffness that may be associated with some chronic pain conditions. So your doctor might instruct you to take paracetamol in addition to other medications to treat the other symptoms. If you take over-the-counter paracetamol regularly for your pain, tell your doctor. It's not advisable to take paracetamol for pain for more than 10 days without your doctor's supervision. It's important to tell your doctor the amount of paracetamol you take on a daily basis.

Some brands of paracetamol contain higher doses of the drug in each pill. These brands' labels may read 'extra-strength', and you should compare the amount of paracetamol various brands contain. In addition, generic forms of the drug are sold widely in pharmacists. Compare prices and the amount of paracetamol contained in brand-name vs generic medicines.

Paracetamol is often combined with other, more powerful analgesics in one medicine. You'll learn more about these drugs later in this chapter.

Common brand names: *Hedex*, *Paracets*, *Panadol*, and many more. *Anadin Extra* and *Disprin Extra* are among the many brands that contain both paracetamol and aspirin. (Consult your pharmacist or doctor to find out more about these medicines.)

Caution: Whilst paracetamol, when taken in the right amounts, shouldn't have side effects, there are some things you should know. It can be dangerous to take paracetamol if you drink alcohol to excess. Government guidelines recommend not more than 14 units per week for women and not more than 21 units per week for men. In addition, the units should be taken through the week, avoiding 'binge' drinking.

If you regularly take more than one or two doses of paracetamol a day, it's recommended that you avoid alcohol because the combined usage can increase your risk of liver or kidney damage. Talk to your doctor about how much and how often you take this drug. He may wish to monitor your liver function or prescribe something else.

It's important to be honest with your doctor about how much beer, wine or spirits you drink on a daily or regular basis. Don't worry about him judging you. Your health is at stake. You might also think about curbing your drinking if you often need to take medicine for pain.

Some brands of pain relievers combine paracetamol with other drugs. Aspirin and ibuprofen, which are discussed further later in this chapter, treat inflammation. If you only need pain relief, you may not need these drugs in addition to the paracetamol.

Non-Steroidal Anti-Inflammatory Drugs (NSAIDs)

All NSAIDs ease pain and inflammation by blocking the production of bodily chemicals called prostaglandins, which also play a role in numerous other bodily functions, including blood clotting, menstrual cramps, labour contractions and kidney function. The specific NSAID your doctor prescribes will depend on a number of factors, including your doctor's familiarity with the drugs and what works best for you.

Adjuvant Therapy

Not all types of pain respond to analgesics alone. Nerve pain and bone pain often require additional treatment with *adjuvant* medications, which are more usually used in other conditions – for example, antidepressants or anticonvulsants. It may seem odd that your doctor prescribes one of these for your pain but he is not implying that you are depressed or are having convulsions, rather that your pain may be treated better by including one of these in your drug regimen.

Antidepressants. Small doses of amitriptyline or imipramine may help your pain control, and may be especially useful at night because they can make you drowsy.

Anticonvulsants. Low doses of clonazepam, carbamazepine or sodium valproate also may help. Another anticonvulsant, gabapentin, is licensed at full doses for the treatment of all types of nerve pain.

Other methods

Heat and Ice. Using heat (hot packs, warm or hot water) and cold (cold water, cold packs or ice packs) treatments, either one or the other or a combination of both, can be very helpful (see p. 158).

TENS. Short for transcutaneous electrical nerve stimulation, TENS can be a useful adjunct to drug treatment in the management of your pain (see p. 147).

Compression and Elevation. When a joint is particularly painful, using an elastic bandage and elevating the joint may be helpful.

Opiates

Some people need an analgesic more powerful than paracetamol alone. Your doctor can prescribe pills that contain paracetamol mixed with stronger drugs for more pain relief. The stronger drugs added are usually opiates. Doctors often prescribe small amounts of opiate drugs; for example, paracetamol combined with codeine or dihydrocodeine for severe, acute (short-term) pain, such as from a broken bone or a herniated (slipped) disc.

Opiates are derived from opium, which comes from poppy seeds. These drugs may also be called narcotics. You may hear the term narcotics and think of junkies, shared needles and illegal drug abuse. Whilst some people illegally abuse opiate drugs, these medicines have great value for people with serious pain. They are safe and effective when you use them according to your doctor's instructions.

For many years, doctors believed that prescribing opiates for people with chronic pain was not a good idea. They felt that people would have to take the drug for a long period of time to maintain pain relief. They also worried that these people would develop a dependence on the drug. (See 'Opiates: Can You Get Hooked?' on p. 70.)

In recent years, newspapers, magazines and TV news programmes have widely reported and discussed celebrities – including TV stars and football players who received prescriptions of the drug following injuries or accidents – who had become addicted to the commonly prescribed opiate drugs. These stories rekindled an old debate about the possible risks of prescribing these drugs for pain. However, they have important, confirmed health value. Most people with severe chronic pain use these prescription drugs properly for effective relief. For these people, these drugs are necessary to live a normal life.

Below are definitions of addiction, dependence and tolerance, all of which can be applied to drugs:

Addiction. A person who is addicted to a substance has a psychological as well as a physical dependence on it.

Physical dependence. A person who stops

Opiates: Can You Get Hooked?

One of the important risks of taking opiates for pain relief is dependence. Dependence on a drug is different from *addiction*. Dependence suggests that the person would experience withdrawal symptoms if they stopped using the drug, whilst addiction is a self-destructive, habitual use of the drug. Abuse of drugs is a serious problem that could be life-threatening.

People who have serious, chronic pain and do not have a previous history of substance abuse are at low risk of developing an addiction to opiate drugs. However, they will develop a physical dependence on the drug; they also might develop a tolerance for the drug, which means that they would require higher and higher doses for pain relief.

The risk of dependence frightens many people with chronic pain, leading them to avoid what could be a very helpful treatment. When it is time to stop taking the drug you can be weaned off it, taking a tapered or gradually lowering dose of the drug.

In addition, some people using opiate drugs may experience reactions of disapproval from friends or family. Such disapproval might make a person uncomfortable about using the drug, or fearful that the drug is somehow dangerous or bad. Opiate analgesics should be safe and effective when used according to your doctor's instructions, just like any other drug.

For some people with chronic pain, other drugs and treatments don't work. If pain has become severe and affects your quality of life or ability to do daily activities, you should discuss opiates with your doctor.

Some doctors don't like to prescribe opiates for chronic pain; others believe that these drugs can provide necessary pain relief and promote better sleep for patients who badly need it. Even doctors who support prescribing opiates for chronic pain agree that they are necessary for only a small portion of patients, and should be used only as part of a wider pain- and disease-management plan. This plan should include other medication options, exercise, healthy diet, lifestyle changes and non-medical pain-relief methods (such as heat and cold therapy or water therapy).

When a doctor and his patient decide that an opiate drug is appropriate, they do so only after the patient understands the risk of dependence and the expected side effects of these drugs.

Why You Might Consider Opiates:

- Opiates are effective medications for managing serious, chronic pain.

- Many people with chronic pain don't need opiates. But those who do should have the option for a trial period.

- The addiction rate from opiates is approximately one per cent. Addiction (compulsive, self-destructive use) is not the same as dependence (withdrawal symptoms if the drug is stopped abruptly).

- Less pain results in increased ability to perform basic daily tasks and could promote better sleep during flare-ups.

Why You Might Avoid Opiates:

- When you use opiates, you treat pain but don't treat the factors that cause it. Therefore, opiates should be used only in the context of a thorough pain-management and disease-management programme.

- Dependence is an expected result of treatment.

- Opiates will dull pain, but not eliminate it. In other words, it isn't a 'cure'.

- Most people develop a tolerance to opiates after a while – from months to years – so they must continue to increase the dosage to have the same level of relief. Along with a higher dosage comes an increased risk of side effects and dependence.

- Opiates have unpleasant side effects such as mental fuzziness, constipation, nausea, drowsiness and itching.

continued on next page

Opiates: Can You Get Hooked? *continued*

- Opiates may not work as well for some types of chronic pain as others. For example, although there have been studies demonstrating the beneficial analgesic effects of opiates in severe osteoarthritis and many other conditions, there have been no studies performed in fibromyalgia.

If you do experience chronic pain that does not respond to other drugs or treatments, you should talk to your doctor about opiates. Discuss the possible risks associated with using the drug. Weigh your feelings about your ability to live an active life with your current levels of pain and your feelings about using these drugs. If you and your doctor decide that opiate pain relievers are an appropriate treatment, follow your doctor's instructions carefully, just as you would with any other drug.

taking the drug will experience withdrawal symptoms. It is not the same as addiction.

Tolerance. Tolerance of a drug is a physical state in which the dose has to be increased over time to produce the same effect, or where the effect of the same dose is reduced over time.

How do opiates work? As we learned in Chapter 1, when a part of your body is damaged or inflamed, your nerve endings send pain signals via the spinal cord to the sensory cortex of the brain, where the sensation of pain is perceived. Opiate drugs interrupt those pain signals, so they never get to the sensory cortex. They cause this interruption by imitating endorphins, naturally produced chemicals that block pain signals.

Common drugs for mild to moderate pain. Weak opiates include codeine, dihydrocodeine and dextropropoxyphene. These drugs are sometimes mixed with paracetamol (e.g. co-codamol 8/500, containing 8 mg of codeine and 500 mg of paracetamol) to treat mild to moderate pain. If pain is more severe, it is better to use these opiates as single ingredient formulations, to avoid exceeding the maximum dose of paracetamol, which can be added separately as required.

Tramadol is a newer synthetic (man-made) opiate.

Caution: Possible side effects of opiate drugs include constipation, weakness or unusual tiredness, lightheadedness or dizziness, drowsiness, nausea or vomiting. These drugs also carry the risk of dependence with long-term use. Drugs containing opiates should not be used with alcohol, as drowsiness, a common side effect of these drugs, could intensify. All these preparations can cause severe constipation. Your doctor might therefore advise you to take a stool softener, fibre supplement, specific foods or a laxative – preferably before constipation has a chance to develop.

Opiate Drugs for Severe Pain

Stronger opiate drugs are available for the treatment of severe pain. These will usually not be necessary to treat the pain of arthritis but may be useful in the event of a severe flare-up or if other drugs have not worked.

Opiate drugs include morphine, oxycodone, fentanyl, buprenorphine and dextromoramide. Some are available as trans-dermal patches (see p. 74) as well as tablets and liquids. You should not stop taking strong opiates suddenly, as this will cause withdrawal symptoms, including restlessness, runny nose, aggressive behaviour, abdominal cramps and alterations in heart rate and blood pressure. If you want to reduce or stop these drugs, talk to your doctor first.

Topical Analgesics

Topical analgesics are creams, ointments, gels, patches or sprays that you apply on the skin over areas where you have pain. These medicines are available over the counter. They may work for a short period of time in small, contained areas of the body, such as your lower back, knee, shoulder or hands. They do not provide long-term relief for pain.

There are two main types of topical analgesics: counter-irritants and NSAIDs.

Counter-irritants contain various oils such as capsaicin (from cayenne peppers), menthol, camphor, wintergreen or eucalyptus. All of

THE SMELL OF PAIN-RELIEF SUCCESS

Some topical analgesics have a very strong scent. This odour may seem unpleasant to you, coworkers, friends or family. In some cases, the relief may be worth the stink! If not, or if you are going to an important event, such as a job interview or a wedding, and don't wish to give off the strong smell, ask your pharmacist to recommend a rub with less or no odour. They can be just as effective.

In addition, some topical analgesics create a strong burning or cooling sensation. If your skin is sensitive, this effect may bother you. If you find the product unpleasant once you have bought it and tried using it, return it to the pharmacy. Or, before you buy a cream, ask your pharmacy if you can open the tube and examine it first.

them work by stimulating the sensory nerves, which compete with the pain signals from the affected area for transmission to higher brain centres and thus close the pain gate. Salicylates and capsaicin cause redness of the skin over the affected area and increase the blood supply, giving a feeling of warmth; menthol and camphor give a cool sensation.

NSAID topical analgesics (e.g. benzydamine, diclofenac, felbinac, ibuprofen, ketoprofen and piroxicam) are formulated for topical administration. They deliver therapeutic levels of drug in the soft tissues and joint fluid without the high blood levels given with oral medications, so there are fewer side effects.

Common brand names: *Algesal, Cremalgin, Cuprofen, Deep Freeze, Deep Heat, Feldene P, Ibugel, Ibuleve, Mentholatum, Movelat, Oruvail, Radian B, Ralgex, Tiger Balm, Voltarol* and more.

Caution: Topical analgesics are available over the counter and seem no different from hand lotion. But they are medicines, and there are some cautions associated with their use. If you are allergic to aspirin, do not use creams containing salicylates, as these could cause an allergic reaction. If you use any topical analgesic, don't use them with heating pads, cold packs or any other type of heat or cold treatment, as you could damage your skin.

Transdermal Patches

Whilst pills are the most common form of pain-relief medication, some people experience problems with medicine taken by mouth. They may encounter side effects, such as severe stomach upset or nausea, or they may have trouble taking the pills at regular intervals. Some people may forget to take the pills at the appropriate time for effective pain relief, and others may have schedules that make it difficult to do so.

For these people or others looking for alternative methods of taking analgesic medica-

tion, one solution may be the *transdermal patch*. 'Transdermal' means through the skin, and these patches contain analgesic medicine (fentanyl or buprenorphene), that is absorbed slowly into the body through your skin. The patch attaches to the skin with an adhesive, almost like a simple sticking plaster. The material that the patch is made of allows the correct amount of medicine to pass into the skin, where it is absorbed into the bloodstream. The duration of the different patches ranges from three to seven days. After that, you remove the patch and replace it with a new one.

Doctors prescribe transdermal patches for people with moderate to severe chronic pain. Most people who use transdermal patches have not found relief through analgesic pills or have some problems taking pills. Whilst the transdermal patch may seem like a pain-relief method you stick on and forget about, these devices contain serious medicine. This medication carries some of the same side effect risks as other opiate analgesics, and you should use the same precautions (such as avoiding alcohol) you would while using other opiates. In addition, external heat sources – such as heating pads or electric blankets – can increase the amount of medicine that is released, causing too much of the drug to enter the body at once. If you use a patch, talk to your doctor about these risks.

We discuss more methods for taking analgesic medicine without using pills in Chapter 6.

FIGHTING INFLAMMATION

One of the causes of chronic pain is inflammation, which is characterized by combinations of redness, pain, heat, swelling and, sometimes, decreased mobility. Inflammation can occur almost anywhere in the body, including on the skin and in the joints, internal organs and soft tissues. Terms ending in the suffix *–itis* indicate inflammation. For example, discitis is an inflammation of a disc of the spine, iritis is an inflammation of the iris in the eye and synovitis is an inflammation of the synovium or lining of the joint capsule. 'Arthritis' is an umbrella term to describe diseases that affect the joints. Although the *–itis* in arthritis implies that there is inflammation of the joints, some types of arthritis, such as osteoarthritis, cause little or no inflammation, just joint damage that can be very painful.

When the body experiences injury or disease, inflammation is part of the body's natural response to the problem, triggering the process of healing and repairing of the damage. Inflammation can be very painful, and in some cases can continue, leading to more damage rather than the body healing itself as it should. That's why in cases of chronic pain that involve inflammation, it's important to reduce this inflammation.

There are a number of drugs that fight inflammation. Some of the most common medicines used to treat this problem are nonsteroidal anti-inflammatory drugs or NSAIDs. You may also see the term 'anti-inflammatories' to describe these drugs. NSAIDs include very common drugs such as aspirin, ibuprofen (*Advil, Brufen, Nurofen*), naproxen (*Naprosyn, Synflex*) or ketoprofen (*Orudis, Ketocid*). As with paracetamol*,* you can buy some medicines containing ibuprofen over the counter (without a doctor's prescription). These drugs may come in generic versions available at your pharmacist's or supermarket. However, other NSAIDs are available only with a prescription. Ibuprofen is available over the counter but also by prescription at higher doses. The higher-dose, prescription versions usually have different brand names from the over-the-counter version. Some brands of medicine combine both NSAIDs (such as aspirin or ibuprofen) and paracetamol to provide both pain relief and an anti-inflammatory action.

There are many different NSAIDs designed to treat the causes of chronic pain. Some medicines are used for a wide variety of problems, but others are used for specific diseases, such as gout or rheumatoid arthritis. (We discuss specific gout drugs later in Chapter 5.) People's tolerance and response to NSAIDs is variable, so if the desired effect is not obtained at the maximum dose of one drug, or if side effects are troublesome, an NSAID from a different chemical class should be tried.

We know that inflammation is the body's response to damage or infection, and that inflammation can be very painful. Untreated inflammation may cause damage to joints and other organs.

How do NSAIDs stop inflammation? NSAIDs work by blocking the enzyme that produces prostaglandins and temporarily stopping their manufacture. This enzyme is called cyclo-oxygenase (COX), and there are two forms: COX-1 and COX-2. It is COX-2 that produces the inflammatory prostaglandins

NSAIDs are commonly used to treat diseases that involve inflammation of muscles, tendons and other soft tissues in the body. These are the soft-tissue rheumatic syndromes, including bursitis (inflammation of a bursa), tendinitis (irritation or inflammation of tendons), carpal tunnel syndrome (where a nerve in the wrist is compressed) or tennis elbow (where the epicondyle, a part of the elbow bone where the muscles attach, is inflamed). They are also used for pain relief in rheumatoid arthritis and osteoarthritis. NSAIDs may reduce swelling and pain during a flare-up of these diseases.

A serious drawback of NSAIDs is that they may cause significant stomach upset or gastrointestinal problems, such as ulcers, particularly if a person uses NSAIDs in high doses or over a long period of time. Serious gastrointestinal bleeding may occur. This risk, and possible counter measures and precautions you can take, are explained in the next section.

Common brands: Diclofenac (*Voltarol*), diclofenac sodium with misoprostol (*Arthrotec*), diflunisal (*Dolobid*), etodolac (*Lodine*), fenoprofen (*Fenopron*), flurbiprofen (*Froben*), ibuprofen (*Advil, Motrin, Brufen*), indometacin (*Indocid*), ketoprofen (*Orudis, Ketocid*), mefenamic acid (*Ponstan*), meloxi-

cam (*Mobic*), nabumetone (*Relifex*), naproxen (*Naprosyn, Synflex*), piroxicam (*Feldene*), sulindac (*Clinoril*).

Salicylates: Aspirin (*Anadin, Aspro, Disprin, Nu-Seals, Phensic*), choline salicylate (*Audax, Dinnefords Teejel*), magnesium salicylate (*Doan's*), salsalate (*Disalcid*), sodium salicylate.

Caution: For all traditional NSAIDs, the side effects are similar. They include abdominal or stomach cramps, pain or discomfort; diarrhoea; dizziness; drowsiness or lightheadedness; headache; heartburn or indigestion; nausea or vomiting. If you notice any severe side effects or if they persist, call your doctor.

NSAIDs and Stomach Problems

Most NSAIDs stop the body from producing all prostaglandins. But not all prostaglandins induce inflammation; some serve good functions, such as protecting your stomach from irritation. So when you stop the body from releasing all prostaglandins, you also keep the good ones from doing their jobs – the lining of your stomach is vulnerable. That's why many people who take NSAIDs over a long period of time or in large amounts for pain wind up with stomach problems. These problems, such as ulcers, can be serious or even deadly. So doctors and researchers have sought ways to offer people pain relief without damaging their stomachs.

Some doctors may prescribe not only an NSAID (see the listing of some commonly prescribed NSAIDs in the previous section) but also a man-made prostaglandin replacement known as misoprostol (*Cytotec*). When the NSAID stops the production of the prostaglandin that protects your stomach along with the one that causes inflammation, this replacement steps in to reduce the chances of irritation. Another drug, *Arthrotec,* combines an NSAID, diclofenac sodium, and misoprostol in a single pill. It's available by prescription only.

Your body also produces an enzyme called COX-1 (COX is short for cyclooxygenase) that produces prostaglandins that help protect your stomach lining from this acid. If your body didn't produce these prostaglandins, the acid would digest your stomach along with the food. That's why NSAIDs, which block the action of COX-1, can lead to stomach damage, particularly in higher doses or when taken for a long period of time. Taking another drug that lessens stomach acid production can reduce your risk of stomach damage.

Another method of protecting your stomach is to combine an NSAID with drugs that lessen stomach acid. Your stomach produces acid through millions of tiny, specialized cells commonly known as acid pumps. The acid pumped out of the cells helps to digest your food, breaking it down in the stomach so it can pass through the digestive system.

There are two kinds of drugs that work to lessen stomach acid production: histamine or H_2 blockers and proton pump inhibitors. H_2 blockers include cimetidine (*Tagamet*), ranitidine hydrochloride (*Zantac*), famotidine (*Pepcid*) and nizatidine (*Axid*). Some of these drugs may sound familiar to you; that's because after many years of being available only by prescription, they are now sold over the counter in lower doses and at a much lower cost.

Proton pump inhibitors are available only by prescription. These medications decrease the amount of acid produced by the millions of acid pumps in your stomach. Proton pump inhibitors are often prescribed for a condition called *acid reflux,* which involves stomach acid moving up into the oesophagus, the tube that leads from your mouth to the stomach. This acid backup causes serious, painful heartburn and *erosions,* or tiny holes in the oesophagus or stomach. Proton pump inhibitors include omeprazole (*Losec*), esomeprazole magnesium (*Nexium*) and lansaprazole (*Zoton*). If taking NSAIDs has caused serious stomach pain or persistent heartburn, ask your doctor whether you should change to a different NSAID, or if one of these drugs may be helpful.

COX-2 Drugs

NSAIDs block the production of both COX-1 and COX-2, and so can lead to severe stomach problems. What if a drug was more selective, blocking only the production of the prostaglandin that causes inflammation and leaving the others alone? Researchers asked themselves the same question, and in 2000 developed a new class of NSAIDs called *COX-2 specific inhibitors* or COX-2 drugs. These drugs selectively stop production of the COX-2 prostaglandin that causes inflammation, but they have much less effect on the

TAKE YOUR MEDICINE (BUT DO IT PROPERLY)

Remember, it's OK to ask a lot of questions about how to take your drugs. In fact, we recommend that you ask as many questions as necessary to understand what you are taking, what effect it will have on your body, and how you should take it. You don't want to take drugs incorrectly. If you do, they might not work, or you might have unpleasant side effects such as an upset stomach.

If you use any drug that your doctor did not suggest or prescribe, even if you follow the label instructions exactly, tell your doctor that you are using these medicines. Just because you don't need a prescription to take a drug doesn't mean that the medicine isn't serious stuff. Any medicine can interact with other treatments you use (even for completely separate health problems other than your pain, such as high blood pressure, allergies or rashes) and cause side effects or damage.

You should also tell your doctor what herbal supplements you may be using. These include glucosamine, chondroitin, St John's wort and many, many more discussed in Chapter 7. These substances may be 'herbal' or 'natural', but they can contain powerful agents that may either interfere with or intensify the action of your drugs. Serious complications, such as bleeding, can occur from drug interactions. Using two treatments containing the same drug might put too much of an active ingredient into your system at once, causing problems. That's why you must tell your doctor everything you are using.

Keep a list of what medicines or other treatments you use, how much you use and how often, and take this list to your doctor. That way, you will be able to remember everything you have done and help your doctor create the most effective pain-management plan for you.

production of COX-1, sparing the protective prostaglandins. These can still do their job, and may reduce your chance of developing ulcers and other serious stomach problems while getting the anti-inflammatory benefits of the drug.

In clinical trials, where drugs are tested on controlled groups of people with the specific health problem the drug is designed to treat, COX-2 drugs caused stomach upset, stomach pain and nausea less frequently than traditional NSAID drugs. Tests on the people who took the COX-2 drugs showed that damage to the *mucus*, or slimy, protective fluid, on the oesophagus was less than with traditional NSAIDs. Normal doses of COX-2 drugs caused two to three times fewer symptoms of ulcers or ulcer-related complications, such as gastrointestinal bleeding or obstruction.

However, the COX-2 drugs have recently been shown to increase the risk of myocardial infarction (heart attack) and stroke, and one, rofecoxib (*Vioxx*) has been withdrawn. There are now clear guidelines for the prescribing of these drugs, including their avoidance in all patients with ischaemic heart disease and atherosclerosis ('furring' up of the arteries). If COX-2 inhibitors are prescribed, they must be used in the lowest possible dose for the shortest possible time.

Common brands: Celecoxib (*Celebrex*), and etoricoxib (*Arcoxia*).

Caution: Same as other NSAIDs (see p. 76), except may carry a reduced risk of stomach damage. COX-2 drugs may not offer the same protection against heart disease that traditional NSAIDs do, so if you do take an NSAID for this purpose, do not use COX-2 drugs.

In the next chapter, we look at more drugs used for treating chronic pain conditions. Most of these drugs treat the condition causing the pain, rather than dulling your perception of pain. Many of these new drugs are the result of groundbreaking medical research conducted in recent years to identify the specific malfunctions in the body that lead to inflammation and pain. These drugs could open a door to a more active life for many people in debilitating chronic pain, a door these people once thought was closed forever.

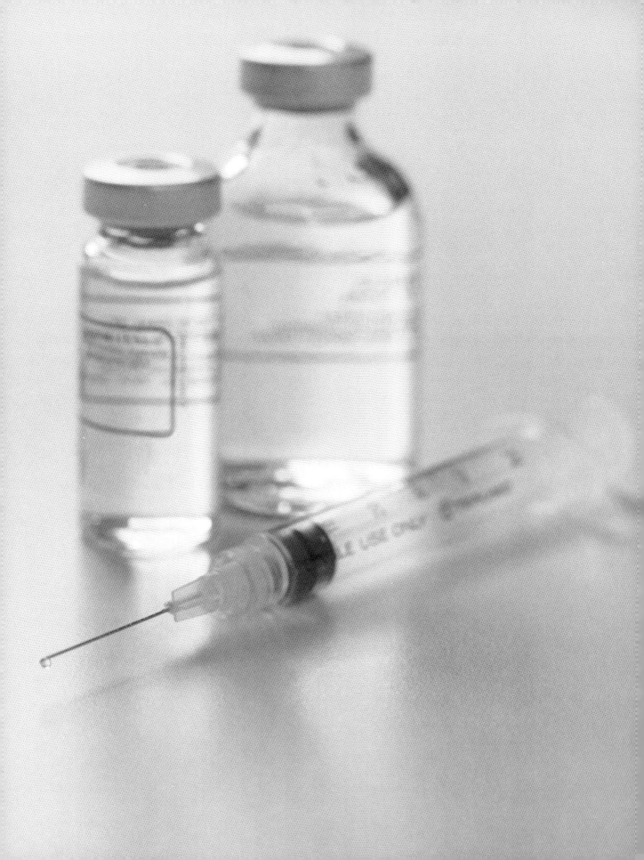

Corticosteroids, DMARDs and More

5

CHAPTER 5:
CORTICOSTEROIDS, DMARDs AND MORE

As we have already discussed, some drugs can treat the underlying cause of your pain, thereby reducing or even eliminating it. The diagnostic process discussed in Chapter 2 will help your doctor pinpoint the cause or causes of your pain. With this information, he can map out a course of treatment, perhaps using some of the drugs discussed in the previous chapter or in this chapter.

In this chapter, we examine some of the drugs that fight disease by helping to correct the malfunctioning processes in the body that can lead to widespread inflammation and pain. We look at some chronic pain syndromes that may need a combination of drugs to treat their many symptoms, and other types of drugs that may reduce pain for many people with chronic problems. We also examine a therapy for knee pain that involves replacing the lubricating fluid often lost in osteoarthritis of the knee.

CORTICOSTEROIDS

Corticosteroids are powerful drugs, available by prescription only, that try to reduce the inflammation associated with some serious forms of arthritis and related diseases that cause intense pain. As we learned in Chapter 2, in diseases such as rheumatoid arthritis, a person's immune system – the system the body uses to defend itself against disease – goes awry. The body's immune system attacks itself, when it should be attacking viruses, bacteria or other organisms that make you ill. It is because the autoantibodies are involved that these conditions are known as autoimmune diseases.

In rheumatoid arthritis, autoantibodies attack your own joints or, sometimes, organs such as the eyes, lungs or skin. The result can be severe inflammation, pain and damage to the joints or organs. To fight this inflammation – which can be disabling in some cases – doctors may prescribe corticosteroids.

These drugs are also known as *glucocorticoids* or *steroids.* Your body makes its own steroids, including cortisol, in the adrenal glands, located above your kidneys. The cortisol your body makes keeps normal internal functions running smoothly. We now have a synthetic but much more powerful steroid similar to cortisol called prednisolone to treat autoimmune diseases such as rheumatoid arthritis, Crohn's disease (a painful disease involving the digestive tract), lupus and many more. This drug helps to dampen down the body's inflammatory response.

In many situations, inflammation is an important part of the immune system's response to infection. The chemical messengers released by the white blood cells may cause local redness and swelling as well as pain and fever, but these all serve a useful purpose. In autoimmune disease, however, the inflammation is not helpful but damaging. So doctors often prescribe corticosteroid drugs to reduce the inflammation and bring the disease under control.

Corticosteroids such as cortisone were considered a miraculous breakthrough when they were discovered and first used to treat rheumatoid arthritis in the late 1940s. The dramatic anti-inflammatory impact of the drugs seemed like the long-awaited 'cure', even earning the scientists who developed the treatment a Nobel Prize for Medicine in 1950. But corticosteroids also may have serious side effects, particularly when used long-term or in high doses. (These side effects are described later in this section.)

Corticosteroids are not merely powerful drugs, but are hormones (chemical messengers) that the body produces. Taking additional corticosteroids through drugs such as prednisolone may lead to considerable side effects and increases the risk of conditions such as osteoporosis (thinning of bones that can lead to serious fractures) and avascular necrosis (death of bone). Corticosteroids slow down the formation of bone, so osteoporosis is a serious risk associated with long-term use of these medications.

Long-term use of corticosteroids, such as in rheumatoid arthritis or other forms of arthritis that involve inflammation, stops the body's adrenal glands (located near the kidneys) from making its own cortisol, one of the body's natural corticosteroids. (Cortisone, the first breakthrough corticosteroid drug, is a man-made version of cortisol.) If a person undergoes unusual trauma, such as an accident or surgery, the body can't produce the boost of cortisol that it needs to recover. Unless the doctor gives extra doses of corticosteroid, the person may collapse and even die. Because of this, it is vital that all patients being treated with corticosteroids carry a warning card with them at all times.

STEROID TREATMENT CARD

I am a patient on STEROID treatment which must not be stopped suddenly.

- If you have been taking this medicine for more than three weeks, the dose should be reduced gradually when you stop taking steroids unless your doctor says otherwise.

- Read the patient information leaflet given with the medicine.

- Always carry this card with you and show it to anyone who treats you (for example, a doctor, nurse, pharmacist or dentist). For one year after you stop the treatment, you must mention that you have taken steroids.

- If you become ill, or if you come into contact with anyone who has an infectious disease, consult your doctor promptly. If you have never had chickenpox, you should avoid close contact with people who have chickenpox or shingles. If you do come into contact with chickenpox, see your doctor urgently.

- Make sure that the information on the card is kept up to date.

Because of the side effects caused by corticosteroids, controversy surrounded the use of these drugs for many years. Until about 20 years ago, many in the medical community advised against using corticosteroids for rheumatoid arthritis treatment except in the most severe cases. That outlook has changed somewhat. Now doctors use these drugs effectively in controlled applications, often in lower doses than used previously for conditions such as rheumatoid arthritis. Some people need a short-term, high (20–60 mg) dose of prednisolone to treat particular conditions or a bad flare of inflammation. Other people respond better to long-term, regular use of a much lower dose of the drugs (such as 2 mg to 7.5 mg per day).

A person who has taken high doses of corticosteroids for more than a few weeks should not suddenly stop taking the drugs. Anyone who abruptly stops taking the drugs may experience confusion, fever, nausea or vomiting, disease flare or even collapse. So it's important to taper the dose gradually while the adrenal glands, which make corticosteroids in the body, build up their capacity to produce normal amounts of cortisol. This process generally takes about two months.

Corticosteroids are usually taken in pill form. For some flares of a painful condition, such as back pain, arthritis affecting one particular joint, bursitis, tendinitis, tennis elbow or carpal tunnel syndrome, doctors may inject corticosteroid drugs through different methods, depending on their pain.

One method is an *intramuscular injection* – injecting corticosteroids into the muscle for absorption into the bloodstream. Two medicines often used for intramuscular injections are triamcinolone (*Kenalog*) and methylprednisolone (*Depo-Medrone*). Some people may be treated with intramuscular injections every two months rather than taking corticosteroids in pill form.

If a single joint is swollen and is extremely painful, a doctor may choose to inject corticosteroids directly into the affected joint. Usually, the doctor removes as much fluid as possible (a process called *aspiration*) before giving the injection. Common joints injected with corticosteroids include knees, ankles, shoulders, elbows, wrists and knuckles.

Joint injections can be very effective at lessening inflammation and pain, because they deliver a much higher concentration of corticosteroid directly to the joint. In addition, joint injections reduce the potential side effects of taking corticosteroids by mouth, because the total dose is much lower. Unlike intramuscular injections, which may be given by any qualified doctor or nurse, joint injections require special training or experience.

Corticosteroid injections may relieve painful flares of tendinitis, bursitis or other soft-tissue rheumatic syndromes. These conditions involve inflammation of the soft tissue near a joint, rather than the components of the joint itself. Doctors can inject corticosteroids in the tissue around the wrist of people with painful carpal tunnel syndrome.

Corticosteroid injections may also be applied at the base of a finger to relieve a 'trigger finger', in which a finger does not unbend normally, but suddenly with a trigger action. In some people who have fibromyalgia, corticosteroids may be injected into *tender points*, areas of great sensitivity and pain.

Some people may find relief through intravenous infusions of corticosteroids (IV therapy). Doctors occasionally administer corticosteroids in very high doses through IV therapy, doses known as *pulses*. (The IV treatment may also be called pulse therapy.)

IV or pulse therapy is effective at pain and inflammation relief, but results are temporary and the natural course of the disease is unchanged. Since the introduction of many other effective treatments in recent years (which we discuss later in this chapter), the use of corticosteroid pulse therapy has declined considerably. However, this treatment may still be effective in certain situations, such as acute flares of pain.

Common Brands: Cortisone, dexamethasone (*Dexsol*), hydrocortisone (*Solu-Cortef, Hydrocortone*), methylprednisolone (*Medrone*), prednisolone (*Deltacortril Enteric*), triamcinolone (*Kenalog*).

Caution: Corticosteroids can have serious side effects: weight gain, puffy face, high blood pressure, lowered resistance to infections. Long-term use of these drugs can increase a person's risk of developing osteoporosis, the dangerous thinning and weakening of bones that can increase the risk of fractures. Long-term or high-dose corticosteroid use can also lead to cataracts, raised blood sugar, insomnia, and mood swings.

Doctors often prescribe corticosteroids in small doses long-term in people with rheumatoid arthritis, limiting many of the side effects of the drugs while still being very effective at controlling inflammation. However, even on these small doses (less than 7.5 mg of prednisolone per day), you will be at risk of a range of infectious diseases. If you come into contact with anyone who has an infectious disease, you should consult your doctor promptly. If you have never had chickenpox, avoid close contact with anyone who has chickenpox or shingles; if you do come into contact with chickenpox, see your doctor as a matter of urgency.

DISEASE-MODIFYING ANTIRHEUMATIC DRUGS

To fight the damaging inflammation present in rheumatoid arthritis, lupus and similar diseases, doctors now use powerful drugs that suppress various malfunctioning body processes and thus slow down or modify the natural course of the disease. These drugs are called disease-modifying antirheumatic drugs, or DMARDs for short. This category includes newly developed, highly targeted and powerful disease-fighting drugs called *biological response modifiers*. We discuss these drugs in detail later in this chapter.

A commonly used DMARD for treating arthritis-related diseases is *methotrexate*. This drug was originally developed in the 1940s for treating leukaemia and breast cancer. In diseases such as rheumatoid arthritis, methotrexate can kill the abnormally behaving cells that lead to joint inflammation, damage and pain. Methotrexate is one of the first drugs that may be used in moderate to severe rheumatoid arthritis.

As with cancer, in rheumatoid arthritis and similar inflammatory forms of arthritis, the abnormal cells involved reproduce and grow at an abnormally fast rate. So the idea of killing these abnormally dividing cells that lead to joint damage and pain makes sense. However, cancer and arthritis are two very different diseases. In cancer, if you kill 99 per cent of the cancerous cells, the remaining 1 per cent will continue to divide and cause disease, eventually returning the person to the same level of illness. But in rheumatoid arthritis, killing most of the abnormal cells can provide great pain relief for the person. Therefore, much lower doses of methotrexate are needed to treat rheumatoid arthritis – often less than one-tenth of that used to treat cancer. That's important, because methotrexate can have serious side effects, including liver damage, increasing susceptibility to infection, mouth sores and hair loss.

Some people with painful, chronic, inflammatory arthritis find relief from long-term, low doses of methotrexate (the typical dose is 7.5 mg once a week, either in a single dose or divided into three given at intervals of 12 hours), only a small percentage of people needing higher doses.

The development of DMARDs was a major breakthrough in the fight against arthritis-related diseases, which can cause serious chronic pain and disability. Like methotrexate, most DMARDs (pronounced DEE-mards) were originally used to treat other serious diseases before being used for rheumatoid arthritis, ankylosing spondylitis, psoriatic arthritis (a painful disease that includes skin rash and joint pain), Crohn's disease and others. But many of these drugs seem to help people who were once felt beyond help, not only easing their pain but also stopping or at least slowing down the damage the disease causes to body parts.

Doctors may prescribe one DMARD or more than one in combination. They may prescribe one DMARD for a time then switch you to another. Why? Every person's disease responds differently to these drugs, and it may take time to find the right drug or combination of drugs for your problem. A decrease in effectiveness with one DMARD could develop, and your doctor would then have to prescribe another drug. In clinical tests, DMARDs have been shown to delay the progression of disease, alter the natural course of the disease, prevent further damage and control chronic pain caused by the disease.

DMARDs are serious, powerful drugs that require frequent monitoring by your doctor, including blood or urine tests (see p. 35). Risks can include liver damage, high blood pressure, increased risk of infections and other potentially life-threatening side effects. Although DMARDs can treat the underlying cause of the disease, if the disease causes inflammation (as diseases such as rheumatoid arthritis and ankylosing spondylitis do), you might need to take an NSAID along with your DMARD.

Ideally, a doctor should prescribe methotrexate or other DMARDs once he determines a diagnosis of rheumatoid arthritis or other disease requiring this type of drug, and before any joint erosions or damage appear on X-rays. Early treatment seems to give the greatest beneficial effect.

With most DMARDs it will take at least six and up to twelve weeks before any benefit is seen. Monitoring for the possible depression of the bone marrow function by regular full blood counts is necessary with most DMARDs.

Common brands: Auranofin or oral gold (*Ridaura*), azathioprine (*Imuran*), ciclosporin (*Neoral, Sandimmun*), hydroxychloroquine sulphate (*Plaquenil*), leflunomide (*Arava*), methotrexate, penicillamine (*Distamine*), sulfasalazine (*Salazopyrin*), sodium aurothiomalate (*Myocrisin*).

Caution: DMARDs may have serious side effects, including rashes, ulcers, diarrhoea, kidney or liver problems, fever, dizziness, nausea or vomiting, pain and more. People using DMARDs may require frequent monitoring by their doctor.

Biological Response Modifiers

Biological response modifiers (or BRMs) are an even newer class of disease-fighting drugs that can treat the malfunctioning body processes that lead to diseases such as rheumatoid arthritis, lupus or Crohn's disease. BRMs target specific chemicals that may be causing unchecked inflammation and suppress their production.

These drugs often provide astonishing levels of relief in some people who had almost lost hope that they would ever experience less pain and increased mobility. The four current BRMs on the market are etanercept (*Enbrel*), infliximab (*Remicade*), anakinra (*Kineret*) and adalimumab (*Humira*). These drugs have passed the clinical trial stage and have been approved for use in selected patients.

How do these drugs work? They inhibit or block the production of *cytokines,* substances in the body's immune system. Cytokines, in normal circumstances, fight disease. In people with autoimmune diseases, the immune system may produce excess cytokines. This unchecked cytokine production may lead to inflammation that in turn leads to pain, joint damage and lost function or mobility. The biological response modifiers etanercept, infliximab and adalimumab work in different ways to stop the production of a cytokine called *tumour necrosis factor,* or TNF, to stop inflammation and, hopefully, prevent further damage. Another biological response modifier, anakinra, blocks another inflammation-causing cytokine called *interleukin-1.*

These drugs cannot repair joint damage that has already occurred. But, for many people, they can reduce inflammation and restore some ability to perform daily functions. Some people who take these drugs experience dramatic relief of pain and improved mobility.

Whilst these drugs are very helpful for many people, biological response modifiers do affect the immune system. Therefore, people using these drugs might be at greater risk of infections. You and your doctor should not begin your BRM therapy during an active infection, and may wish to modify your dose if you develop an infection of some kind. If you develop an infection while receiving this therapy, you should notify your doctor immediately to receive treatment for it.

The National Institute for Health and Clinical Excellence (NICE) has recommended that etanercept, infliximab and adalimumab be used only in patients who have failed to respond to at least two DMARDs. They should be withdrawn after three months if no response is seen.

Anakinra is currently licensed in the UK but is not recommended for routine treatment.

Etanercept and adalimumab are given by injection. Etanercept is injected twice weekly in 25 mg doses, underneath the skin in the thigh, abdomen or upper arm.

Adalimumab can be used in combination with methotrexate or other DMARDs.

Infliximab is given by an intravenous (IV) infusion, either at a hospital or at an outpatient clinic. This is a two-hour procedure. The dose is based on your body weight, usually between 200 and 400 mg per dose. The first dose is repeated at 2 and 6 weeks, then given once every 8 weeks after that. Infliximab is approved only for use in combination with methotrexate at this time.

Common brands: Adalimumab (*Humira*), anakinra (*Kineret*), etanercept (*Enbrel*), infliximab (*Remicade*).

Caution: When you are taking any of these drugs, your doctor will monitor your progress and reactions to the drug. You may experience irritation or redness around the place of the injection or IV needle insertion. Serious infections have been reported in some patients using TNF-blockers.

With etanercept, you may also experience pain or burning in the throat or a stuffy nose, as if you had a cold. With infliximab, you may experience abdominal pain, cough, dizziness, headache, muscle pain, nasal congestion or runny nose, nausea, shortness of breath, sore throat, tightness in the chest, unusual tiredness, vomiting or wheezing.

OTHER DRUGS FOR CHRONIC PAIN

Some chronic pain conditions may require specific drugs that address pain and the cause of the pain. In addition, some drugs developed to treat disorders not related to pain – such as seizures or irregular heartbeat – may have some pain-relief benefits as well.

Gout Drugs

Gout, which we learned about in Chapter 1, is a disease caused by a build-up of uric acid crystals in the body. There are a number of drugs that can either help reduce the uric acid build-up or help your body flush out the uric acid more effectively.

Gout is very painful. People experiencing a gout flare may not be able to walk on the affected limb, keeping them from work and other daily activities. A joint affected by gout can be swollen, red and extremely sensitive to any touch (even a mild breeze). Gout attacks can happen suddenly, and should be treated immediately. If gout persists or recurs over a long time, a person might develop *tophi,* or solidified deposits of uric acid crystal. Tophi are firm, swollen nodules that can appear under the skin, often visible externally, in the fingers, toes or other areas.

Gout is one of the few chronic pain conditions that can be linked to diet, although this is not the only factor that plays a role in the development of gout. People with gout should avoid certain foods that are high in purines and should watch their consumption of alcohol. This dietary plan may help lower the amount of uric acid in the person's body and lessen the risk of a gout attack. In addition, drinking at least two litres of water or other non-alcoholic, non-caffeinated beverages every day will help the person's kidneys flush the uric acid out of the body so that it does not build up and form crystals. Attacks of painful gout can be prevented.

If you have a gout attack, it's important to treat the pain and inflammation quickly to obtain relief. Because gout is an inflammation of the joint, an anti-inflammatory drug is used. Whilst your doctor may prescribe one of the NSAIDs listed on p. 75, another anti-inflammatory drug, colchicine, can relieve the symptoms of the gout flare, such as swelling and pain. Aspirin should never be used as an analgesic in an acute attack.

It is vital that treatment with preventative agents is not begun until any acute attack of gout is over because, otherwise, they could prolong the symptoms as well as making them worse.

You can treat the underlying cause of the disease using one of several effective drugs. Some people naturally produce too much uric acid, leading to the build-up that causes gout. For these people, a drug called allopurinol (*Zyloric*) slows the body's production of uric acid. Other people with gout don't excrete uric acid efficiently, so it builds up in the body. For these people, the drugs sulfinpyrazone (*Anturan*) and probenecid (*Benuryl, Probecid*) help increase the amount of uric acid flushed out by urination.

Common brands: Allopurinol (*Zyloric*), colchicine, probenecid (*Benuryl, Probecid*), sulfinpyrazone (*Anturan*).

Caution: Drugs may have various side effects, including skin rash, itching, diarrhoea, nausea or vomiting, stomach pain, headache and more. Some of these drugs may interfere with other drugs you take for unrelated health problems, so discuss your other medications with your doctor.

Drugs for Fibromyalgia

Fibromyalgia, which we also learned about in Chapter 1, includes various symptoms, such as widespread muscle pain and tenderness in various points throughout the body. Some people with fibromyalgia experience debilitating pain and sensitivity to the slightest touch or pressure. These symptoms can ruin a person's ability to live a normal life or work. People with fibromyalgia often also have extreme fatigue and sleep problems, creating a vicious cycle. They hurt, so they can't sleep; they can't sleep, so their body can't re-energize itself.

Why does this happen? It's hard to say. But we know that your body must have deep, restorative sleep – known as *REM sleep* or delta sleep – in order to restore itself and function well the next day. Some studies suggest that people with fibromyalgia sleep but do not sleep deeply or long enough. Because they do not get the proper amount of REM sleep, their bodies do not restore themselves and they feel achey, fatigued and irritable the next day.

The medical community has recognized fibromyalgia for only the past 20 years or so – and there are still medical professionals who do not recognize the disease – and little is known about why fibromyalgia occurs or how to treat it effectively with drugs.

At present, the only drugs used to treat fibromyalgia are drugs currently approved and used for other health disorders. However, many effective drugs used to treat rheumatoid arthritis, for example, were used originally to treat other diseases such as cancer. So existing drugs can be useful for treating fibromyalgia while research for new, fibromyalgia-specific drugs continues.

Researchers believe that one possible cause of fibromyalgia is that the person produces too much substance P (see p. 12), although the reason for this overproduction is unknown. Too much substance P might intensify the person's response to pain, causing them to perceive normal touches or pressures as painful.

People with fibromyalgia might also have an abnormal production of serotonin, a chemical that regulates the way the brain controls pain and moods. Some research has found that people with fibromyalgia either have low amounts of serotonin or process serotonin poorly. Not having enough serotonin may cause poor sleep, one of the most common symptoms of fibromyalgia.

Decreased serotonin production may also lead to a change in the way substance P is produced or released in people with fibromyalgia. For them, when a pain stimulus occurs, the decreased serotonin levels cause the pain messages travelling to the brain to become more intense or pronounced than the stimulus – such as a light touch – would merit. So someone with fibromyalgia would perceive something that might not cause pain in most people as very painful.

Despite continuing research, there is currently no definitive evidence pointing to what causes fibromyalgia. So there are no drugs available to treat the root cause of the disease. Doctors can only treat the symptoms with other drugs and hope that the person finds some relief.

Antidepressants and anti-anxiety medicines, prescribed in low doses, can help the person with fibromyalgia to sleep better. This group of medicines includes tricyclic antidepressants and selective serotonin reuptake inhibitors (SSRIs).

In addition, muscle relaxants might ease the muscle tension and pain common in fibromyalgia, and also promote sleep. Gentle sleep medications can also help the person with fibromyalgia get a restful night's sleep, allowing them to restore their energy and feel better the next day.

Many people with fibromyalgia take an analgesic for their pain. If you have fibromyalgia, you should ask your doctor if regular doses of an analgesic such as paracetamol would be helpful and safe for you. NSAIDs are not recomended because they aren't effective in fibromyalgia and can have unwanted side effects.

Another treatment option for chronic fibromyalgia pain is the newer, opiate drug tramadol. This drug might relieve pain for people who do not achieve adequate relief from antidepressants. People with fibromyalgia may wish to take the analgesics in addition to their other medications rather than in place of them.

Talk frankly and openly with your doctor about your pain and what options exist to relieve it. All drugs can have serious side effects if used improperly or unnecessarily, so trust his judgement.

One of the main goals of doctors treating fibromyalgia is to promote deep, restorative sleep. The most effective drugs now available for this purpose are the tricyclic antidepressants. In addition, the use of another kind of

antidepressant, selective serotonin reuptake inhibitors (SSRIs), might be taken along with tricyclics.

In addition, some people with fibromyalgia may find that the *anticonvulsant* medicine gabapentin (*Neurontin*) may ease the leg pain, tingling sensations or numbness that can be a symptom of fibromyalgia. See the section on anticonvulsants on p. 92.

Common brands: Tricyclic antidepressants: amitriptyline hydrochloride, doxepin (*Sinequan*), nortriptyline (*Allegron*)

SSRI antidepressants: citalopram (*Cipramil*), fluoxetine (*Prozac*), paroxetine (*Seroxat*), sertraline (*Lustral*)

Anticonvulsants: gabapentin (*Neurontin*), pregabalin (*Lyrica*).

Caution: For all tricyclic antidepressants, possible side effects can include constipation, dizziness, drowsiness, dry mouth, headache, tiredness and weight gain. There are numerous possible side effects for other types of antidepressants, including decrease in sexual desire or ability, drowsiness, anxiety or nervousness, dry mouth, gastrointestinal problems and more. Using alcohol along with many antidepressants can increase the effects of drowsiness or cause other problems. Ask your doctor or pharmacist for a complete list of side effects or cautions.

Other Drugs

There are a number of other drugs that your doctor might prescribe for pain relief. Some of the most common are skeletal muscle relaxants, which we touched on briefly in the previous section. These drugs help to relax tensed, painful muscles in any part of the body. Doctors may prescribe them to treat conditions such as back or neck pain, temporomandibular (jaw hinge) joint disorder, fibromyalgia and more.

Muscle relaxants act on the central nervous system to send messages to the muscles to lessen their tension or spasm, which helps to relieve pain. Muscle relaxants can also make you feel sleepy or drowsy, which may be helpful if your pain has kept you from sleeping. These drugs should be used short-term, not as a long-term treatment.

Common brands: Carisoprodol (*Carisoma*), orphenadrine (*Biorphen, Disipal*).

Caution: Muscle relaxants can make you feel sleepy or drowsy, and this effect can be more intense if the drugs are taken by someone also using alcohol or taking central nervous system depressants (which include antihistamine drugs, prescription analgesics or opiates, and sleeping medicines) or some tricyclic antidepressants. These drugs may cause blurred vision or clumsiness in some people, so use caution. It's probably best not to drive or operate any machinery while you are taking these drugs.

Gabapentin (*Neurontin*) and pregabalin (*Lyrica*) are anticonvulsant drugs used to control seizures in people with epilepsy. But they are sometimes prescribed for other uses, including easing neuropathic pain. Neuropathic pain may be caused by damage to the nerves themselves or be related to diseases such as multiple sclerosis, diabetes or a painful

skin condition called shingles which is caused by the same virus that causes chickenpox. Some types of chronic back pain are neuropathic. Whilst gabapentin usually doesn't have side effects, there is a risk of drowsiness, headache, fatigue, blurred vision, tremors (shaking of the limbs), anxiety or irregular eye movements in some people. Pregabalin is said to have a lower incidence of these effects.

Central pain syndrome is a very painful chronic condition that develops after damage to the central nervous system, such as after a stroke or an injury, or due to the disease multiple sclerosis. People with neuropathic pain often describe it as shooting, burning or stabbing. Movement, changes in temperature and other unrelated stimuli may aggravate the symptoms. People with central pain syndrome often find some relief with gabapentin or nortriptyline.

Common brands: Gabapentin (*Neurontin*) and pregabalin (*Lyrica*).

Caution: Dizziness, drowsiness, headaches, loss of coordination, nausea.

Other anticonvulsants that may be prescribed for jabbing-type pain are carbamazepine (*Tegretol*) and phenytoin (*Epanutin*). Another drug that may be used for relief of pain is mexiletine (*Mexitil*), an antiarrythmic drug used to treat irregular heartbeats. Mexiletine may be used to relieve burning-type pain associated with neuropathic pain. Side effects of mexiletine may include dizziness, nausea, vomiting, tremor causing difficulty walking or shaking hands. In a very small percentage of patients, a continuous infusion or intravenous application of an anaesthetic such as lidocaine may be prescribed. Such an application can only take place in a pain clinic.

Common brands: Carbamazepine (*Tegretol*)

Caution: Upset stomach, drowsiness, vomiting, loss of appetite, diarrhoea, hallucinations, insomnia, irritability, mental confusion, headache, dry mouth, speech problems, coordination problems, impotence, mouth and tongue irritation. Do not eat grapefruit or drink grapefruit juice one hour before or two hours after taking carbamazepine.

Common brand: Phenytoin (*Epanutin*)

Caution: Upset stomach, drowsiness, redness, irritation, bleeding, swelling of the gums, vomiting, constipation, stomach pain, loss of taste, loss of appetite, weight loss, difficulty swallowing, mental confusion, blurred or double vision, insomnia, nervousness, muscle twitching, headache, increased hair growth.

Common brand: Mexiletine (*Mexitil*)

Caution: Dizziness, nausea, vomiting, tremor causing shaking hands or difficulty walking.

In the next chapter, we examine some other medical methods for treating pain, including some that involve surgical treatments and high-tech devices implanted in your body to offer continuous pain relief.

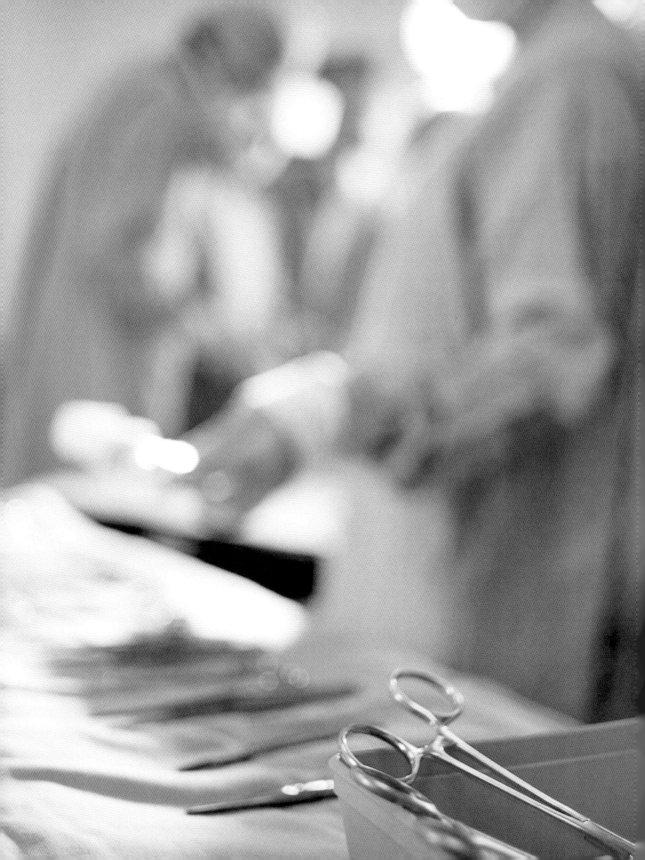

Pumps, Implants, Surgery and More

6

CHAPTER 6:
PUMPS, IMPLANTS, SURGERY AND MORE

Chronic pain can interfere with every aspect of your life. When you are in constant pain, everything becomes very difficult: work, recreation, sex, taking care of your family, household tasks, taking care of yourself. So finding the right pain-relief method is very important.

For many people, the medications discussed in the previous chapters – mostly taken by mouth in the form of pills – may not provide enough relief. In addition, these people may find that their GP runs out of solutions when it comes to their pain treatment, requiring a referral to a doctor specializing in pain treatment. Whether or not you need to go to a pain clinic, your chronic pain may require treatment that goes beyond swallowing daily pills. Today's technology offers some new methods of delivering pain medication and inflammation-fighting drugs to the source of your pain.

Hopefully, one of the many pain-relief medicines or techniques will work to help control your pain. Remember, using a multi-pronged approach – trying different medical, complementary and psychological methods as part of a comprehensive pain-management plan – may be the best way to deal with pain. Chronic pain may be constant, but, with help, there's a good chance you can keep it under control so that you can get on with your life.

INJECTIONS AND IMPLANTS

The most common pain-relief treatments described in the previous two chapters are, primarily, taken by mouth. The medicine in these preparations is digested in the stomach and absorbed into the bloodstream. There, it flows throughout the body and the active ingredients go to work. Analgesics can work at different levels of the process that makes us feel pain. Some work at peripheral pain receptors (nociceptors) and others work at the level of the spinal cord, altering the transmission of pain signals to the brain, or higher, in the central nervous system.

In some cases, it may be more effective to put a concentrated dose of medicine directly into the source of pain or injury – into a muscle, joint or nerve. Doctors do this by giving injections, or by placing implants within the body that release medication at a steady rate. Injections and implants may administer analgesics, anaesthetic (or numbing) medicine, corticosteroids or a combination.

Injections

Injections can send a high dose of analgesic medicine directly into the body, by-passing the digestive system and so delivering pain relief more quickly. However, their effects may not last as long as those of oral medications (another term for pills that you swallow). For long-term pain relief or disease management, oral medications are preferable.

However, certain pain-relieving techniques may provide additional pain relief for many people who have not found adequate relief through traditional drug treatments or non-drug therapies, such as heat or cold, or exercise. These include: injections directly into an affected joint, bursa or trigger point; nerve-blocking injections of peripheral nerves; and injections into the spaces around the spinal cord, including epidural and spinal techniques.

Injection therapy has a range of side effects. Some people experience side effects from the medication itself, such as corticosteroids (see p. 82). Other complications include the risk of infection from the injection or problems associated with the medicine leaking into the surrounding tissue after it is injected.

There is also the risk that the doctor – usually a rheumatologist, orthopaedic surgeon or anaesthetist – may place the needle in the wrong spot. This could cause a puncture or rupture of a tendon, nerve, blood vessel or the surrounding structures. Also, the drug can be injected into the wrong place, which may have other unwanted effects.

Viscosupplementation

Some people with the chronic pain of knee osteoarthritis – a very common, often debilitating condition – get relief from viscosupplementation. In osteoarthritis of the knee, some people experience a breakdown in production of the sticky, elastic fluid that helps cushion and protect the moving parts of the joint. When this happens, the cartilage in the knee is unprotected and can deteriorate. When cartilage deteriorates, the person can experience painful, bone-on-bone rubbing when he or she moves the knee, such as in walking, bending or climbing stairs. This pain can be severe, making it difficult for the person to carry out normal activities.

Viscosupplementation improves the viscosity (thickness) of the synovial (joint) fluid, decreases pain and swelling of the joint, and increases the depth of the cartilage covering the bone.

Viscosupplementation can be achieved in two ways. One is by taking supplements of glucosamine and chondroitin daily, and the other is by having injections of hyaluronic acid directly into the joint.

Glucosamine and Chondroitin

With glucosamine – which is available as either glucosamine sulphate or glucosamine hydrochloride – the dose is vital: it must be 1,500 mg (maximum) per day. This can be taken all at once or, perhaps better, divided into three doses of 500 mg. The beneficial effects will not be seen for one to two weeks. The amount for chondroitin is 1,200 mg per day in divided doses. The benefits are not generally seen for one to two months.

The US National Institutes of Health (NIH) is running a placebo-controlled double-blind study to see whether combining glucosamine and chondroitin will achieve better results than either supplement alone.

As with any supplement or remedy, always discuss the matter with your doctor before starting any nutritional supplement.

Injections of Hyaluronic Acid

Injections of hyaluronic acid must be performed by a rheumatologist or an orthopaedic surgeon. There are three preparations for use in this way: *Hyalgan*, *Synvec* and *Ostenil*. The injections are given weekly for three to five weeks.

With any of these products, a local anaesthetic, or numbing agent, may be applied to ease the pain or discomfort of the actual injection. In addition, before injecting the hyaluronic acid, your doctor may drain and remove fluid from the joint capsule to make room for the more viscous injected fluid.

Viscosupplementation may relieve pain for a number of months. Doctors often suggest that people limit vigorous physical activity (such as sports or hiking) for one or two days after the injection.

Other than pain at the site of the injection, which may be relieved by giving an anaesthetic first, and joint infection, which is rare, viscosupplementation carries few side effects. However, some people should not use these products. People with any allergic reactions to hyaluronan preparations, or with allergies to bird feathers, eggs and/or poultry should not use hyaluronic acid therapy.

Corticosteroid Injections

Injecting a corticosteroid (steroid) preparation directly into the inflamed area allows your doctor to deliver a high concentration of drug to the problem area. The rest of your body is not exposed to the effect of the corticosteroid because only small doses are used. Corticosteroid injections are used in the treatment of rheumatoid arthritis, gout, and other inflammatory conditions such as bursitis and tendinitis.

Corticosteroid injections do carry risks – repeated use in the same area can cause thinning and weakening of the tissues. Bleeding into the treated area and infection are rare complications.

Sometimes, corticosteroid injections are used alone; for example, in bursitis. Or they may be part of a treatment programme including anti-inflammatory medications and physiotherapy; for example, in rheumatoid arthritis.

The beneficial effects are a reduction of swelling and pain. Improvement usually takes place within one to two days, and lasts for from a few weeks to several months. Joints commonly treated are the knee, hip, shoulder, elbow, and the facet and sacroiliac joints of the spine.

Sometimes, a local anaesthetic drug is mixed in with the corticosteroid medicine. This anaesthetic can provide almost immediate, temporary, pain relief to the affected area while the corticosteroid takes effect.

With any type of joint injection, doctors usually advise you to rest or limit your use of the joint for 24 to 48 hours after the injection. This rest period helps prevent leaking of the injected fluid, and also helps the medicine reduce the inflammation that may be causing pain. How long you may have to rest really depends on your situation. Your doctor will advise you.

Corticosteroids can also be injected directly into a painful bursa if you have bursitis in any of the 150 bursae in your body. The most common sites of bursitis are the shoulder, hip, buttock and elbow. Bursae cushion the areas in the joints where bones meet muscles or tendons. When they become inflamed, moving the joint becomes very painful. Doctors can inject a dose of corticosteroids into the area to reduce the bursa inflammation, lessen the pain and restore mobility to the joint.

Trigger point injections. Trigger points are areas where muscles or *fascia* (fibrous tissues beneath your skin) are sensitive and painful. These trigger points can be treated by injecting a combination of local anaesthetic, to numb the area, and corticosteroid medication, to reduce inflammation and swelling. This can provide pain relief and improve mobility. Trigger point injections take between 5 and 15 minutes and may involve between one and five injections. The treatment can take three to four days to take effect, but it can have long-term positive results in relieving pain. In severe cases, injections of botulinum toxin (*Botox*) can be used to achieve longer-lasting relief.

Nerve Block Injections

Nerve blocks are performed by injecting a small amount of local anaesthetic around the nerve that supplies the painful area. This gives effective pain relief, but it may be of relatively short duration. The technique may be useful in helping to diagnose the cause of your pain. Sometimes a corticosteroid is added to the local anaesthetic, as this may help the block to last longer. If the nerve block is repeated several times, some patients notice a significant reduction in their pain that lasts longer than would be expected. This may be due to an effect in the dorsal horn of the spinal cord.

There are a number of possible complications with nerve blocks. They include: failing to produce a block; infection, which is prevented by performing the blocks in the sterile environment of an operating theatre; bleeding, which is more likely in certain areas than others; and misplacement of the injection, which can be prevented by using X-ray guidance.

There are three main types of nerve block injections: peripheral, spinal and sympathetic.

- **Peripheral nerve blocks** are simply injections of anaesthetic around the nerve to reduce sensation and pain. This type of nerve block injection might be done in smaller, concentrated areas of pain, such as in the ankle or elbow.

- **Epidural nerve blocks** are used for pain that affects wider areas of the body, such as your leg or back. In this type of nerve block, the doctor injects anaesthetic medicine near the spinal cord. You may have heard about *epidural injections*. Epidurals are used to relieve severe pain in large areas of the body.

They can be performed at any level of the spine, from the lumbar region up to the neck. Epidural blocks are used commonly in childbirth, making labour much easier on mothers. But doctors are also using epidural injections to relieve severe back pain, such as sciatica, a common and often debilitating problem. Complications of the epidural technique are rare, but, when they do occur, they can be serious. They include severe headache (1–2 per cent), infection (less than 1 per cent) and, very rarely, temporary paralysis.

- **Sympathetic spinal nerve block injections** are another type of pain-relief injection that is used to control pain arising from the sympathetic nervous system. This system is a network of nerves that control basic life functions such as blood pressure, heart rate and body temperature. People with the disease *reflex sympathetic dystrophy*, sometimes known as *complex regional pain syndrome,* may be experiencing pain due to damage or disruption in normal activity of these nerves. Doctors use sympathetic spinal nerve blocks as part of the regimen to relieve pain from this type of disease.

All of these procedures are performed in hospital, often as a day case, so you can be home and resting a few hours after your procedure.

SURGICAL PAIN-RELIEF PROCEDURES

People with serious chronic pain may not obtain sufficient pain relief from options such as drugs or complementary therapies, and find that surgery is the next step. Surgery can be a beneficial treatment for extreme chronic pain but must be considered carefully.

Many people with arthritis have joint surgery, such as arthroplasty or total joint replacements, as a way to remove damaged, painful joints and restore mobility. In other cases, surgeons can treat neuropathic pain through implantation devices or specific nerve operations designed to treat the source of severe pain. Joint and bone operations are performed by orthopaedic surgeons, while nerve operations are performed by neurosurgeons.

All of these procedures require major surgery, a hospital stay, lengthy recovery and rehabilitation and, often, significant cost.

Some surgical procedures produce amazing results. A person with a severely damaged joint due to osteoarthritis or rheumatoid arthritis can find, after joint replacement surgery and recovery, that their pain is reduced and their mobility is greatly restored. Other people find that surgery is not as effective, or serves only as a partial treatment for their serious pain.

Some of the most common forms of surgery used to treat arthritis pain are outlined in the following sections.

Arthroplasty or Total Joint Replacement

Arthroplasty, or total joint replacement, involves removing damaged joints and replacing them with a new joint component made of metal, ceramic or plastic. Many thousands of joints are replaced annually, the most common being the hips, knees, shoulders, elbows, fingers and knuckles.

The surgeon secures the new, artificial joint with either special bone cement or through a cementless procedure where the body's tissues and bone grow slowly around the joint to hold it in place. Arthroplasty requires weeks of recovery and rehabilitation. Some new surgical techniques for joint replacements are less invasive, requiring a smaller incision and shorter recovery time after surgery. In addition, there are new, higher-flexibility knee replacements that allow greater range of movement. You can expect your new joint to last for ten to fifteen years, after which you may need a further replacement.

Arthroscopy

Arthroscopy (see p. 41) may be used as a diagnostic procedure to determine the cause of joint pain, although magnetic resonance imaging (MRI) has largely taken over. However, arthroscopy is used to perform many different surgical procedures without having to make a large incision. This can make recovery much faster.

Some surgeons use arthroscopy to treat minor damage to cartilage, bones, ligaments or tendons that may be causing pain. Arthroscopy procedures are most often done on knees and shoulders. Doctors use the arthroscope to view the damage to joints, and then may trim ragged cartilage or remove loose bits of tissue that may be causing discomfort or pain.

The advantage of arthroscopic surgery is that it requires less anaesthesia and less cutting than a standard operation. It is often done on an outpatient basis, eliminating the need for a hospital stay. Furthermore, patients recover from arthroscopy much more quickly than they do from some other types of surgery, and they can get back to normal activities more quickly.

Although arthroscopy is used most often on the knee or shoulder, increasingly it is being used to treat damage found in other joints affected by injury or arthritis, such as the elbow, hip, wrist and ankle.

Other Operations

Osteotomy. Osteotomy is the cutting and reshaping of bone that may be deformed or out of alignment, leading to wear of one part of the joint, causing pain and impaired movement. By changing the way the bones of the joint fit together, particularly the knees, the weight of the body is redistributed over the whole surface of the joint.

Arthrodesis. In arthrodesis (also called bone fusion), the surgeon cuts the bones of the arthritis-damaged joint and fuses the ends of the bones together, holding them with a pin or rod that is inserted into the bones. This procedure creates a more stable, but rather immobile, joint. However, it may reduce pain and increase a person's ability to move around, although not to bend the joint as he once could.

Arthrodesis is often used for joints that aren't commonly replaced with prostheses. It is effective for people who, for reasons such as joint infections or poor bone quality, aren't good candidates for total joint replacement surgery.

Resection. Resection involves removing a portion of the bone from a stiff or immobile joint, which creates a space between the bone and the joint. Although the bone itself never grows back, more flexible scar tissue fills the space and offers more flexibility. However, the joint is less stable. Resection is most common in upper extremities, such as the wrist, thumb or elbow, and in the foot.

Synovectomy. In synovectomy, the surgeon removes damaged parts of the synovium, or joint lining, which can become inflamed and painful in some forms of arthritis. Usually, the surgeon can perform a synovectomy using an arthroscope, requiring a less invasive operation and shorter recovery time. Synovectomy is not always a permanent solution: sometimes the diseased synovium grows back, requiring another synovectomy or perhaps joint replacement.

For more information on many types of joint surgery, read one of the booklets produced by the Arthritis Research Campaign (ARC; contact details in the Resources section), which cover the most common types of joint surgery, explain the procedures, and prepare you for surgery, recovery and rehabilitation.

Nerve-Related Operations

For neuropathic (nerve-related) pain, neuro-surgeons can perform different operations to treat the pain at its source: the damaged or inflamed nerves. We have already learned about nerve blocks, but here are a few more of the most common procedures to treat neuro-pathic pain:

- **Neurectomy** (including peripheral neurec-tomy) is a procedure to remove the dam-aged peripheral nerve that is causing pain.

- In **spinal dorsal rhizotomy**, usually reserved for severe chronic pain or cancer-related pain, the surgeon carefully cuts the roots of one or more of the damaged nerves that radiates from the spine, or the nerve root where a painful condition is occurring. Other rhizotomy procedures include cranial rhizotomy, selective rhizotomy and trigemi-nal rhizotomy.

- **Sympathectomy** or **sympathetic blockade** describes a procedure in which the surgeon injects a drug, usually guanethidine, into the affected area to eliminate pain in a specific area, such as an arm or leg. People with reflex sympathetic dystrophy syn-drome or other conditions (e.g. renal colic, pancreatitis) may undergo this procedure.

- **Deep brain stimulation** or **intracerebral stimulation** is a very new and extreme form of internal nerve treatment involving surgi-cal stimulation of the thalamus portion of the brain. This treatment usually is reserved for people with serious neuropathic pain, such as central pain syndrome, and is rarely performed.

Is Surgery the Right Option?

As you consider whether to have surgery, keep in mind that every person's situation is different. You may not benefit from the same surgery that a friend, family member or the majority of participants in a medical study did. Your doctor may advise against a particular operation or warn you that its chances of success are low. Even if your doctor thinks that surgery can help you, there are many factors that both you and your doctor must consider, including the following:

- **Other health problems.** If you have heart disease or lung disease, the strain of some types of surgery may be too much for you. Before having any kind of surgery, it's important to have other health problems under control.

- **Your medications.** In some cases, you may need to stop some of the medications you are taking for a while before surgery. For example, such drugs as aspirin and other non-steroidal anti-inflammatory drugs, which you may be taking to ease pain and inflammation, may interfere with blood clotting and cause you to bleed excessively during surgery. On the other hand, corticosteroid medications, such as prednisolone, may be needed at larger doses during surgery. The reason is that these drugs are similar to hormones our bodies produce naturally in response to stress. In people

who take synthetic corticosteroids, the body's ability to increase its own production of these hormones may be hampered. Therefore, additional medication may be necessary to help your body meet the demands of the situation.

- **Infections.** If you have any type of bacterial infection in your body, even a tooth abscess, you'll need to have it cleared up before you undergo any surgery. One possible problem after joint surgery is infection, which can spread from another part of your body to your joint through the bloodstream.

- **Your weight.** If you are overweight, it's best to start losing weight before you decide to have surgery. Being overweight may put extra stress on your heart and lungs during surgery. If you are undergoing knee- or hip-replacement surgery, excess weight can be stressful on a prosthetic joint component. For any surgery involving a weight-bearing joint, excess body weight can make rehabilitation more difficult by placing strain on the joint and making it more difficult to do the exercises needed to make the joint stronger after surgery.

- **Strength and fitness.** Although any rehabilitation programme after surgery will involve exercises to strengthen the muscles around the affected joint, doing such exercises beforehand may increase your odds of surgical success. Similarly, aerobic exercise can prepare your heart and lungs for the rigors of surgery and rehabilitation. To learn more about what you can do to improve your physical fitness before surgery, consult your doctor or a physiotherapist.

- **Your care as you recuperate.** One of your major concerns as you consider surgery may be caring for yourself in the days and weeks that follow. Things to consider include: Who will care for your home, children, pets or plants while you are in the hospital? Who will care for you once you are home? Depending on the type of surgery you have, it may be a few days or a couple of months before you are able to do such things as stand for prolonged periods, drive a car, vacuum or shower without the assistance of another adult. Consider your personal support systems – or the possibility of getting someone to help you for a while – before the operation.

If you prepare properly for surgery, you'll have less to do or be concerned about when the time arrives, and relieving yourself of that stress now may help you recuperate faster. Nevertheless, recovering from surgery – particularly major surgery, such as total joint replacement or resection – requires a commitment. The amount of work you put into a recovery process often makes the difference between success and failure and your risk of adverse effects. In general, here's what you can expect to do following major joint surgery:

- **Wear support stockings.** Immediately after surgery and until you are up and moving, your doctor will want you to wear tight, elasticated stockings on your lower legs to prevent blood clots from forming in them. Blood clots, which can break loose and clog the lungs, are among the most common and dangerous complications of joint replacement surgery.

- **Work your muscles.** Following surgery, and maybe even before, your doctor will probably refer you to a physiotherapist who will give you a programme of exercises that help strengthen the muscles that support the joint. It's important that you follow the programme faithfully, even when it may be painful to do so, to gain as much use of the joint as possible. Exercise will begin gradually and become progressively more strenuous as your joint gains strength and mobility.

- **Protect your joints.** Immediately after replacement surgery of the knee or hip, and for about six weeks after surgery, you'll need support when you walk. At first, you'll use a walking frame, and later you'll graduate to a walking stick. You may need to wear a brace on the joint and use special, strategically placed pillows when you lie down.

Protecting a joint after surgery is important, regardless of the type of surgery you have. Your doctor, surgeon, nurse and physiotherapist will give you advice on joint protection.

- **Heed limits.** As you start to feel better, you may be tempted to do too much too soon. Resist this temptation. Using your joint more than it's ready to be used or moving the joint beyond its intended range of motion can cause damage and possibly necessitate further surgery.

Be sure to do all the exercises your doctor and physiotherapist recommend, but also be sure to know and heed your joint's limits. If you have any doubt as to whether an activity is safe, consult your doctor.

- **Take your medications.** It's important that you take any medications your doctor prescribes exactly as directed. Medications you may need following surgery include opiate analgesics to relieve pain and make it easier to perform your exercises; blood thinners to reduce the risk of blood clots; antibiotics to reduce infection risk; and, of course, any medications you need for your arthritis control, including any NSAIDs, corticosteroids or DMARDs that you usually take. Although the joint on which you had surgery will soon feel better, unfortunately, the surgery will not slow damage or inflammation to other joints.

- **Steer clear of infection.** Even after you've recovered from surgery, it's important that you take extra precautions against bacterial infection if you have a joint prosthesis (or any type of implant in your body). For example, if you cut your finger on a kitchen knife or step on a nail, it's important that you do not let the wound become infected. There is the possibility that any infection that enters the body through the bloodstream may settle in the joint, causing prob-

lems that might require further surgery to correct. If you need to have any dental treatment done, let your dentist know that you have an artificial joint, so that extra precautions can be taken if necessary.

By preparing for joint surgery and following doctors' orders and common sense afterwards, the operation may offer a lifetime of pain relief and increased mobility. As with any operation, however, joint surgery offers no guarantees. In rare instances, joint surgery results in infection, which requires further treatment or surgery. Prostheses have a limited life expectancy in even the best of circumstances, so if you have joint replacement as a young adult or in middle age, there's a chance that the prosthesis will loosen and have to be replaced in time.

Because surgery may be less successful the second, or third, time around, and most people don't want to face the prospect of another operation, age may be a major factor in your decision to have a joint replaced. Fortunately, there are many medications and other measures that can delay or eliminate the need for joint surgery. For those who do undergo joint replacement, advances in materials and surgical techniques are making the procedure work better and the joints last longer.

Anaesthesia: to Sleep or Not to Sleep

Regardless of the type of surgery you have, it's almost a certainty that you will need some type of anaesthesia. While most people associate anaesthesia only with pain relief, it has an additional purpose in the operating room – it allows the surgical team to control a wide range of natural bodily reflexes, such as heart rate and blood pressure, that could fluctuate dangerously in response to the trauma of surgery.

Your surgeon will recommend one of three types of anaesthesia – general, regional or local – to block your pain and control your natural bodily reflexes.

General Anaesthesia. General anaesthesia temporarily stops the brain's overall ability to sense and remember pain. Under general anaesthesia, usually a mix of inhaled and intravenous drugs, you are asleep.

Local or Regional Anaesthesia. With both local and regional anaesthesia, you are fully aware of what is going on during the operation and will remember it. With local anaesthesia, the anaesthetist blocks the pain signal where the nerve begins. For minor surgery on the foot, for example, you might have a few localized injections that will numb just the foot.

For more complex knee surgery, on the other hand, the anaesthetist might block pain responses from entire lower regions of the body by injecting an anaesthetic into the outer covering of the spinal column (called *epidural anaesthesia*).

With epidural anaesthesia, you have full feeling in your upper body and will be able to speak with the surgical staff during the actual procedure.

Which Anaesthesia Is Best? The best anaesthesia will depend on a number of factors, including your general health, the procedure you are having and personal preference. A local or regional anaesthetic generally is less risky and you recover from it more quickly.

General anaesthesia is often necessary for long, complicated operations. Even so, doctors often use regional anaesthesia for such procedures as some joint replacement. Doing so may enable to you to be up and active more quickly, which may improve the odds of long-term success of the procedure.

IMPLANTABLE DEVICES

Another relatively new option for people who do not get enough relief from traditional methods are implantable devices, tiny machines that pump prescribed amounts of analgesic medicine directly into the space around the spinal cord to relieve pain. This treatment is sometimes known as *intrathecal drug therapy*. This type of therapy is used for people with severe chronic pain or pain associated with nerve damage that does not respond to typical oral drugs.

Neurostimulators are another kind of implantable device that use electrical impulses instead of analgesics to block pain signals from reaching the brain. Neurostimulation is sometimes used for people with nerve damage or neuropathic pain.

Before being considered for these devices, a patient must have received a proper trial of oral analgesic therapy *plus* a trial of all other pain interventions (such as acupuncture, TENS (see p. 147), epidural blocks, nerve blocks and surgery). Only when all this has failed to provide adequate pain relief would an implant be considered.

Both types of implants require you to have surgery and, in many cases, a short hospital stay. The procedure to implant and activate the device lasts about one to two hours.

Intrathecal Drug Delivery Pumps

Before considering you for this treatment, your doctor will perform a test or trial run of the implant using a temporary catheter attached to a pump that is outside your body. This test typically lasts for about seven days. It allows you and your doctor to see how effective the treatment will be, and how much your abilities to move around or perform daily tasks improve. This is important because having the procedure carries risks; as well as the usual possible risks from surgery and general anaesthesia, there is the possibility of the device being misplaced or of an infection developing. Also, the pumps are expensive (about £20,000).

If this produces good pain relief, your doctor must surgically implant a pump about the size of your palm that releases a continuous dose of analgesic medication (usually morphine) directly into the intrathecal space around the spinal cord. The intrathecal space is where pain messages are most effectively interrupted. Through a catheter – a slender, flexible delivery tube – the pump delivers the medicine to this space. The pump is set by your doctor to release medicine at a particular rate (the dose depends on your level of pain).

Because the spinal cord is the body's telephone line for pain messages, blocking or interrupting the transmission of the messages helps relieve pain. The pump device is usually inserted through an incision in the lower abdomen, or near where your belt sits on your body.

Implantable pain-relief devices involve risks and it's very important to place the device properly.

For people with severe, chronic pain, these devices can be very effective and offer a number of advantages. The pumps release medicine automatically into the body, which means you don't have to remember to take pills on a schedule. Moreover, the devices release the drug at regular intervals, giving a continuous stream of pain-relieving medication.

In addition, you will experience fewer side effects, such as nausea or grogginess, from implantable devices than from taking pills. This is because intrathecal pumps can often relieve pain with much lower doses of medicine than would be required by a person taking analgesics in pill form. However, it is likely that you will still need to take oral preparations for your pain, as the pump rarely provides complete relief of pain.

There are risks to any kind of treatment. Implants or pumps, partly because they involve surgery, do carry risks. These risks include allergic reactions to the medicine, bleeding, problems with the device or improper implantation, headaches, injuries to the spinal cord, paralysis or infections from the implantation. The devices may leak or shift, or even fail to work, requiring additional surgery. People with implanted devices must see their doctor regularly to refill the medicine in the pump (required about every three months) and to make sure it is running properly.

Neurostimulation Devices

Another useful type of implanted device uses electricity, rather than analgesic drugs, to relieve pain. This technique, called *spinal cord stimulation* or *implanted neurostimulation*, involves delivery of electrical impulses to one of the major nerves (a nerve root) emerging from the spinal cord, through a tiny wire, placed carefully inside the body. The impulses stimulate the nerves to interrupt the pain signal transmission.

As with intrathecal pain therapy, your doctor will consider this procedure only if a proper trial of all other treatments, including surgery, has failed. The procedure involves surgery. A surgeon will implant a tiny device, called an electrode or a lead, near your spinal cord. The lead is a special, flexible, insulated wire designed for medical use. The lead and another small device called a neurostimulator send electrical impulses to the spinal cord to block pain signals from reaching the brain.

The neurostimulator is powered either by an implanted battery (known as a fully implanted neurostimulation system) or an external power source (known as a radiofrequency system). With the fully implanted system, the battery power source and all the wiring are inside your body. With the external power source, you will have a small antenna attached to your skin with adhesive, and you must carry a battery pack, which looks like a small TV remote control or personal pager.

With neurostimulation therapy, your pain is replaced by a tingling sensation.

Another type of neurostimulation method is *peripheral nerve stimulation*, in which the surgeon places the lead near the specific peripheral nerve that is damaged and causing pain. (See p. 9 for more on the peripheral nerves.) Peripheral nerve stimulation uses only the external radiofrequency system for power.

As with intrathecal pumps, you will need to have a trial run of a neurostimulation device. This is to ensure that the lead is sited over the correct nerve and that you obtain adequate pain relief without experiencing any unpleasant or unbearable sensations. The trial period usually lasts a few days. You and your doctor will test and monitor your response to the device. If it works properly and your pain is reduced by more than 50 per cent, you'll undergo a short operation to implant the device, followed by a brief hospital stay.

If neurostimulation seems like an option you might be interested in, it's important to talk to your doctor about the risks and cautions. The impulses may be uncomfortable, feeling like electrical shocks or jolts. Some people may develop an infection related to the surgery or a *haematoma* (a big bruise, or collection of blood). Other possible complications include movement or disconnection of the lead, and battery failure (it usually lasts for three to six years). Because these devices are very expensive, you will be carefully assessed before your doctor goes ahead.

If you have an electronic implant in your body, outside electronic devices such as power tools or airport security scanners might interfere with your neurostimulator. You should ask your doctor about any risks and what precautions you should take to prevent problems. There may be some activities you should avoid while using your neurostimulator. You will be taught how to adjust the power of your neurostimulator if you notice unpleasant jolts or sensations or if a stronger degree of stimulation is needed.

fiNDING WHAT'S RIGHT FOR YOU

With any pain-relieving medications or devices, there are side effects, risks and cautions. In addition, some people may find that the drug or device may simply fail to relieve their pain. In these cases, doctors sometimes say this person has *intractable pain,* meaning that their pain has not responded to any treatment available. If your pain has not responded to the medical treatments you have tried, there may be other options for finding relief: complementary therapies. We discuss these therapies in the next chapter.

Even if drugs or devices do provide some pain relief, you may find that incorporating complementary therapies and lifestyle changes (such as adopting an exercise plan or changing your diet) can help you better manage your pain and overall health. In addition, they may help you cope better with your chronic pain and the disease that causes it.

For people with chronic pain, developing a plan for coping is essential. Some pain clinics offer guidance in coping with chronic pain, so if there is one in your area, ask your doctor if you can be referred. Pain-management programmes and the Expert Patients Programme are discussed in Chapter 2. Arthritis Care also runs training courses to help people of all ages to be in control of their arthritis.

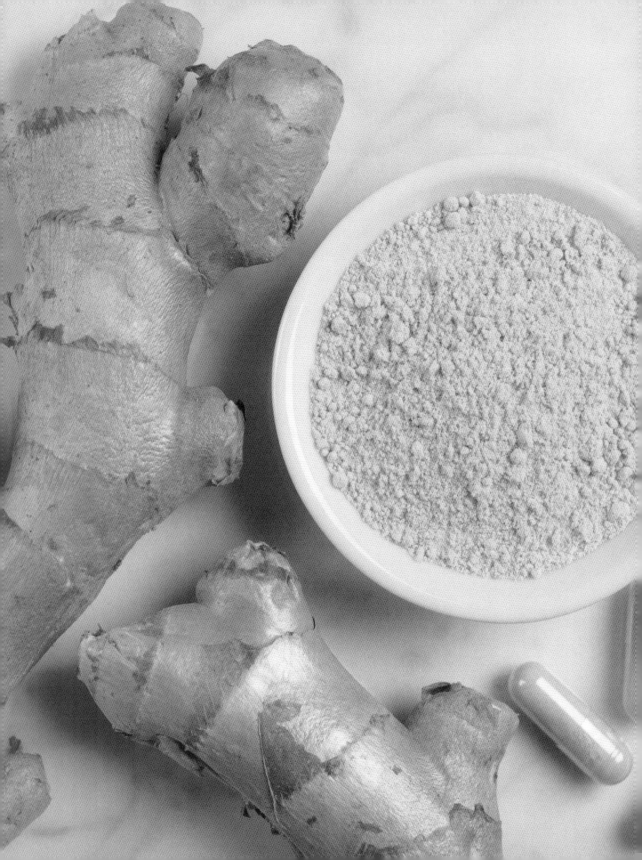

Natural Options:
Herbs, Supplements
and More

7

CHAPTER 7: NATURAL OPTIONS: HERBS, SUPPLEMENTS AND MORE

Most people with chronic pain wish they could find relief in a simple pill. But for most people with arthritis, fibromyalgia, chronic back problems or other painful conditions, controlling pain on a daily basis means trying a variety of techniques and strategies.

These strategies can include drugs, lifestyle or habit changes, and complementary therapies as part of the pain-management plan that you create with your doctor's supervision. With your doctor's help, you can identify which therapies are most effective for you and which therapies to avoid.

If you have chronic pain, you've probably read magazine articles or heard friends talk about complementary therapies. Also called *alternative* therapies or *natural medicine*, this category of treatments contains many different types of pain-relief options. Some of these alternatives involve the help of a *practitioner* or professional trained or skilled in administering these therapies. Other strategies are things you may try on your own.

There are some controversies associated with complementary therapies and their use. There are few studies to support the efficacy of most of these therapies. Yet some may be quite beneficial for pain relief for some people. One possible source of information and advice is your doctor, who may will be able to discuss alternative options for pain relief and steer you toward treatments that are more

likely to work. Other good sources of reliable information are Arthritis Care (and similar reputable self-help organizations) and the Arthritis Research Campaign.

An important point to remember is that other types of therapy that you try should be *complementary* – that is, in addition to or alongside – and not *alternative* – that is, instead of – the treatment prescribed by your doctor.

Note. If you are taking any medication that is considered critical – such as insulin – or that has narrow limits for dosage – such as warfarin – you should avoid using herbal products or nutritional supplements. *Always* talk to your doctor or pharmacist first.

Let's learn more about the differences between complementary and 'orthodox' medical treatments, and why some treatments may fall somewhere between the two.

WHAT IS COMPLEMENTARY THERAPY?

Complementary therapy is a loose, umbrella term for a group of treatments that fall outside the standard (orthodox) medical therapies prescribed by doctors. Medical therapies include drugs, surgery, physiotherapy, occupational therapy and any treatment supervised by a medical doctor or physio- or occupational therapist. Whatever is left – and this category includes a wide variety of treatments

– may be considered complementary. However, some complementary therapies are offered by GPs or at GPs' surgeries; for example, acupuncture and homoeopathy.

The terminology can be confusing. Some people call therapies such as acupuncture or herbal supplements 'traditional medicine' because people have been using these therapies for centuries. Yet we now refer to drugs and surgery as 'traditional medicine' or 'allopathic medicine' and call herbs, acupuncture or other non-medical treatments 'complementary.'

Whilst some medical doctors once ignored complementary therapies as either bogus or inadvisable, many now accept their use by patients and discuss these treatments as part of an overall pain-management plan. Some doctors even practise *integrative medicine,* a blend of mainstream medical treatments and complementary or natural therapies, which has been championed by the Prince's Foundation for Integrated Health.

Many people consider complementary therapies safer because they are more 'natural'. Yet many of these treatments have side effects or risks. Some natural treatments contain an active ingredient also found in a mainstream medication. If you take both, you could receive a dangerous excess of that ingredient.

The line between drugs and natural treatments is not so clear. In fact, the first drugs for treating pain came from natural sources, such as opium poppies (opiate analgesics), willow tree bark (aspirin and other salicylate NSAIDs) and others. For centuries, doctors offered their patients these preparations to relieve pain and treat other symptoms. Over time, scientists refined these substances or discovered ways to make them more effective. Even now, scientists work constantly to make safer and more effective drugs. Some drugs are synthetic versions of chemicals your body produces naturally – for example, hormones such as insulin and corticosteroids.

Still, some people feel uncomfortable using a lot of drugs to treat their pain. They believe that taking a lot of 'chemicals' is 'unnatural' and not as healthy as using treatments that seem closer to their natural state. Some people may be frustrated by the lack of pain relief offered by their drugs, so they turn to complementary treatments in the hope that they will be more effective. Complementary treatments, like over-the-counter drugs, don't require a prescription, so a person in pain can just go to the shop, read labels and buy whatever they want to try. Whilst this seems easier than going to your doctor, it can also be a dangerous game.

The possible dangers are:

- overdose of a constituent of the complementary therapy also being taken in a mainstream drug

- contamination of the complementary treatment with undisclosed active ingredients

- stopping taking the mainstream treatment

- interaction between the complementary treatment and the mainstream drugs

We discuss these more fully later, in the section 'Evaluating Complementary Therapies'.

No matter what complementary therapy you try, it's very important first to discuss what you want to use with your doctor. These 'natural therapies' can be very powerful medicines or treatments. They may also interfere with the drugs your doctor has prescribed. So talk to your doctor about complementary therapies. He may be able to suggest complementary treatments that will be effective for relieving your pain. He also will help you avoid therapies that will interfere with your current medications or those that don't work at all.

What's the Controversy About Complementary Therapies?

In the past, many medical doctors were sceptical of complementary therapies. These therapies were untested by scientists and did not have to go through the stringent assessments of the Committee on Safety of Medicines, an independent advisory committee that advises the UK Licensing Authority on the quality, efficacy and safety of medicines. If you wished to try any complementary treatment, you did so at your own risk and without any guidance or approval from your doctor, pharmacist or reputable organizations and government agencies that regulate health treatments.

These days, more and more people are using complementary treatments and purchasing products and services that fall into this category. This trend has awakened many established government and medical institutions. They are beginning to look more closely and seriously at complementary therapies.

Respected universities and medical research institutions now conduct scientific studies on these therapies to see if they are safe and effective for patients to use.

In 2000, the House of Lords Science and Technology Committee recommended changes to the regulation and development of complementary therapies. These included the recommendation that all complementary therapies should be assessed with the same rigour as is required of conventional (orthodox) medicine. Despite this, currently less than 1 per cent of all medical research funding is spent on studies of complementary therapies.

There is still much we do not know about complementary therapies. When you use them, you do so at your own risk. By talking to your doctor and/or pharmacist before trying a complementary treatment, you can at least get the professional opinion of someone you know and trust. When you're in pain, you may be willing to try anything in the hope of finding relief. But you don't want to try something that will do more harm than good, and you don't want to waste your time and money on treatments that may do nothing at all.

Drugs and other medical treatments go through a very serious, lengthy process of testing and retesting to determine their effectiveness and possible risks of their use. Once the Committee on Safety of Medicines approves medications, doctors may prescribe them, but even then, continued studies and examinations track any possible problems associated with the drugs' use.

Evaluating Complementary Therapies

If you are in pain, you may be willing to try anything to find relief. You will see hundreds of magazine ads, infomercials and Internet banner ads that tout various products or devices for pain relief. You may hear your friends talk about amazing new treatments that work better than drugs, with no side effects. You may pick up bottles of herbal supplements at the supermarket, pharmacy or health-food shop with labels that claim astonishing pain relief and restoration of mobility, strength and energy – all available to you by taking a simple pill.

If you're considering any complementary treatment, do your homework first. Don't assume that a product is safe just because the label or advertising says it's 'natural'. Remember: hemlock, the deadly poison, is natural, too.

Here are some useful guidelines to follow as you consider trying complementary treatments:

- **Know the facts about the therapy.** Although drugs and other medical treatments are monitored and regulated by government agencies, complementary therapies do not have to undergo that type of scrutiny to be marketed to the public.

- **Buyer beware.** If a product or a practitioner (such as an acupuncturist or chiropractor) makes unrealistic claims, such as 'It will cure your disease', be wary. If a practitioner suggests that you discontinue your conventional medical treatments, consider it a strong warning that something is not right. Most reputable practitioners work in conjunction with your medical treatment, understanding that their therapy is just one part of your total pain-management plan.

- **Do your own research.** Read up on any complementary therapies you wish to try. Many books and web sites are devoted to topics related to complementary therapies. Ask your doctor if he has any knowledge of the treatment. Four good sources of information about common complementary treatments are Arthritis Care's booklets *Drugs and Complementary Therapies* and *Food for Thought* (discusses supplements), the Arthritis Research Campaign booklet *Complementary Therapies and Arthritis* and the Consumers Association's *Which? Guide to Complementary Therapies* by Helen Barnet.

Evaluating Complementary Therapies *continued*

- **Search the Internet.** There are numerous web sites devoted to information about complementary therapies for chronic pain and other conditions. However, some may provide unsubstantiated information, some may exist mainly to sell you products and some may be biased toward a particular health philosophy. You will have to use your own judgement about the validity of the information you collect online. If you are not sure where to look, start with reliable sources such as government web sites and those of Arthritis Care, the Arthritis Foundation of Ireland, the Arthritis Research Campaign (ARC) and the Coventry Pain Clinic, and see what information they give and the links they offer to other organizations. Contact details are given in the Resources section.

- **Be a healthy sceptic.** Just as you would be sceptical when buying a gadget for your car or your home, be sceptical where your health is concerned. Avoid treatments that claim to work by a secret formula, or to be a magical cure or miraculous break-through.

  Whilst important treatments may be found in nature or outside the laboratory, if they really work well, the chances are they won't be secret for long! Be wary of products that are advertised only in the backs of magazines, through phone marketing or through direct mail. Reputable treatments will be reported in medical journals and picked up by the mainstream press. How manufacturers verify the product's claims is important as well – if the product has only testimonials as proof that it works, rather than scientific studies, be wary.

- **Talk openly with your doctor.** Tell your doctor about any treatment you use, whether complementary, conventional or over-the-counter. Your doctor knows a great deal about the many pain-relief treatments available. He can talk to you about possible side effects and negative interactions with drugs you may be taking. Your doctor should work with you to oversee your pain-management plan and decide what new therapies are of possible benefit.

- **Watch out for high price tags.** Some complementary treatments can be expensive. Find out the charges for treatment sessions and how many you will need, as well as the cost of remedies and how much you will need to take. Compare the costs of various treatments and decide what options offer the most pain relief for the money.

- **Find a reputable practitioner.** If you do use a complementary treatment, seek out a qualified professional practitioner. Find out about professional societies that provide certification for these treatments and ask for a list (see the Resources section).

- **Don't abandon a treatment that works.** If you do try a complementary treatment for pain, don't stop taking your prescribed drugs. This could cause problems or interrupt your pain relief, or both. Talk to your doctor to make sure this treatment is safe to use with your prescribed drugs.

- **Don't mix and match.** Be cautious about potential interactions between your drugs, both prescription and over-the-counter, and any herbal medicines or treatments you try. Ask your doctor or pharmacist before adding any natural or herbal treatment to your pain-management plan. Even something that seems harmless may affect the way your prescribed treatments work.

Some complementary therapies have undergone scientific, controlled studies by reputable institutions such as universities, but many have not undergone any scientific study at all. No official approval is necessary for them to be sold to the public. In this chapter, we also discuss some unproven remedies and some treatments that probably don't do anything to relieve your pain.

In recent years, the government and the medical establishment have taken comple-mentary therapies more seriously, and scientists are beginning to study complementary therapies for effectiveness and safety. Still, there is no governmental regulation of most of these therapies, so it's important for you to be a wise consumer when experimenting. The guidelines in this chapter offer some steps you may wish to take to find the most effective treatments.

A big risk associated with trying complementary treatments without a doctor's advice is that you may not be getting what you paid for. Because herbs, nutritional supplements and other natural remedies available in health-food shops, supermarkets and pharmacists are not regulated, nor required to undergo a rigorous approval process, there's no guarantee that the remedy will be effective or safe despite label claims. There is no guarantee that the remedy contains the ingredients or the amount of the ingredient listed on the label. You could be wasting your time, money and patience. Moreover, it may contain something potentially dangerous that is not disclosed.

If you do purchase herbs, supplements or natural remedies, ask your doctor or pharmacist to recommend particular brands that are more reputable. Don't rely on the advice of friends or unqualified, unlicensed staff in health-food stores or even pharmacies.

HERBS AND SUPPLEMENTS FOR CHRONIC PAIN

When most people think of complementary therapies, they think of herbs, vitamins and supplements, also known as nutritional or natural supplements. These items seem very much like drugs. They often come in pill, capsule, liquid or ointment form and are sold in many 'drugstores'. Most people have good feelings about taking vitamins, herbs, minerals or natural-based compounds, because using something 'natural' suggests promotion of good health.

In the past, these items (other than vitamins and minerals) were found only in health-food shops or sold through mail-order catalogues. But supplements are now available in many other places, including pharmacist's shops and supermarkets. They are advertised everywhere, promoted and sold over the Internet and through direct-marketing networks.

More and more studies are being conducted on herbs, vitamins and supplements to determine their *efficacy* (whether or not they actually work) and safety for humans. There are different types of studies performed on drugs as well as supplements. Studies performed in a laboratory are known as *in vitro* (Latin for 'in glass', as in a test tube), and studies performed on animals or humans are known as *in vivo* (Latin for 'in life'). Reliable scientific studies should be performed under controlled circumstances. In other words, two groups of similar people selected according to specific criteria (such as their age, disease, level of pain) should be tested. One group would receive the supplement to be tested, and the other group would receive a placebo, or fake supplement. (See the box on p. 119 about the 'placebo effect'.) The most reliable tests are 'blind' studies, where none of the participants knows whether they are receiving the real treatment or the placebo.

We don't have a great deal of scientific data to say whether or not most of these supplements work. Many have possible side effects or cautions associated with their use, and you and your doctor should discuss whether you should try them or not. In many cases, it may be safe to use these supplements as part of your pain-management plan, but there's no

THE PLACEBO EFFECT

Before a drug is licensed to be used to treat people, it is thoroughly tested to make sure that it does what it is meant to do and that it is safe. If there is already a drug treatment available, the new one may be tested against the established one: one group of people will be given the established drug and another group will be given the new drug to see whether it is more effective than the other. Neither group knows which drug they are taking.

Another procedure is to test the new drug against a *placebo* – placebo being a Latin word meaning 'I will please'. The placebo is a dummy drug, a pill containing just sugar or some other neutral substance. If people taking the placebo believe that it contains medicine, they might believe that they will benefit from it – the so-called *placebo effect*. The test here is to see whether the new drug is more effective than the dummy drug, which will produce some benefit because the people taking it will expect it.

The most reliable tests are those called 'double-blind' – neither the people giving the drugs nor the people taking them know what is being dispensed. So there is no possibility of bias in the reports. Both groups are monitored carefully throughout the test period so that, if anyone experiences serious side effects, they can drop out of the trial or, if necessary, the trial can be halted.

The placebo effect is always considered when testing the effectiveness of a treatment. Studies have found that as many as 30 to 35 per cent of people receiving placebos report some initial relief from symptoms. However, pain usually returns for most of these people.

This doesn't mean that we should toss out all of our prescription medicines and just eat sugar pills. The placebo effect has to do with the power of the mind to heal, and that's very important and real. Using your mind to help you cope with symptoms and even reduce your sensation of pain is a good strategy that we discuss more in Chapter 8. But most people who sense improvement from a placebo in a trial will probably start feeling their pain again soon. That's because they haven't taken anything for the pain that will really address the physical process behind the pain.

guarantee they will work. It could be a 'may not help, but can't really hurt' situation, so the decision to use them or not is up to you.

Many people report having used some type of dietary or nutritional supplement in the recent past. Because supplements are widely available and easy to use, it's no wonder they are so popular for people seeking pain relief.

However, there are still some concerns. Do these supplements do what they claim to do? Are they safe to use? If the claims for a product seem too good to be true, be very wary!

Below are some commonly used supplements for treating chronic pain, fatigue and inflammation. **Note:** if you are pregnant or breastfeeding, you should not take any of these supplements.

Glucosamine and Chondroitin Sulfate

If you have arthritis or any type of joint pain, you've probably heard of glucosamine and chondroitin sulfate. The market is full of different brands of these popular supplements, and the media has covered the reports of their effectiveness in the news.

Both glucosamine and chondroitin sulfate come in various forms depending on the preparation and brand: capsules, tablets, liquid or powder. Glucosamine (available as glucosamine sulfate or glucosamine hydrochloride) is made from the shells of crustaceans (shrimp, lobster and/or crab), and chondroitin sulfate is made from the tracheas (windpipes) of cattle or pork byproducts.

Both are made from animal products, but they are similar to the material that makes up human cartilage.

Glucosamine and chondroitin are found in human cartilage. Cartilage is the rubbery, flexible material covering the ends of your bones that allows you to move your joints freely and comfortably. Cartilage cushions bones where they meet at joints.

When people develop osteoarthritis, their cartilage often deteriorates. It is believed that supplements such as glucosamine and chondroitin help to repair or restore that cartilage, easing movement and reducing pain. These supplements may relieve pain in people with osteoarthritis on a similar scale with NSAIDs, although they may take much longer to take effect.

Glucosamine may help the body grow, repair or retain cartilage in the body's joints. It also helps cartilage absorb water, lubricating the joint so it moves more easily. Studies on glucosamine have been promising; two recent studies found that the supplement did relieve pain and improve movement function.

Chondroitin is believed to reduce pain and improve joint function by helping collagen (the main component of cartilage) absorb the impact of joint movement better. It may also block the deteriorating action of certain enzymes in the body that may break down cartilage. But there is no current proof that chondroitin stops or reverses the loss of cartilage in the body, as some users believe.

The major study by the US National Institutes of Health (NIH) on both supplements (both separately and in combination) in people with knee osteoarthritis found some benefit only in people with moderate to severe arthritis. Otherwise, over all, there was no benefit

Possible cautions or side effects of chondroitin: Apart from the possibility of diarrhoea, constipation and abdominal pain, side effects are rare, and there are no reports of problems after long-term use. People who also take blood-thinning medications such as NSAIDs might see an increased risk of bleeding if they also take chondroitin.

Possible cautions or side effects of glucosamine: Mild stomach upset, nausea, heartburn, diarrhoea, constipation and increased blood glucose. If you have diabetes, talk to your doctor before trying glucosamine. If you are allergic to shellfish, avoid using glucosamine, because these supplements are made from their shells.

Boswellia

Boswellia, also known as Indian frankincense, frankincense or salai guggal, is a supplement derived from the bark of the Boswellia tree (*Boswellia serrata*) found in India, North Africa and parts of the Middle East. Boswellia comes in capsule or pill form, and the supplement supposedly reduces inflammation and treats various symptoms of painful diseases such as osteoarthritis, rheumatoid arthritis and bursitis.

Possible side effects: Diarrhoea, nausea or rash.

Bromelain

Made from pineapples, bromelain is an enzyme in the tropical fruit's juice that breaks down protein. It's available in tablet form. Bromelain is meant to decrease pain in arthritis and increase joint mobility.

Some evidence supports the claim that bromelain and other protein-dissolving enzymes can relieve pain and inflammation much as NSAIDs do. And bromelain is probably quite safe to use. It may therefore be a good supplement to your overall pain-management plan. In addition, bromelain may help reduce swelling after surgery or injury, which might decrease discomfort.

Possible side effects: Stomach upset and diarrhoea. Bromelain may increase the effect of blood-thinning medicines.

Cat's Claw

Cat's claw is a supplement made from the dried root bark of a vine (*Uncaria tomentosa*) found wild in the Amazon region of Peru. The vine's claw-shaped thorns give the supplement its name. It's sold in capsule, tablet or tea bag (which must be steeped in hot water) form.

Cat's claw vine has been used as a treatment for inflammation and pain in bones or joints for many years, and some people with knee osteoarthritis use the supplement to reduce inflammation and pain. At least one study on animals shows that cat's claw may prevent inflammation and other cell damage.

Possible side effects: Headache, dizziness and vomiting.

Cetyl Myristoleate (CMO)

CMO comes from a waxy substance found in animals. Available in pill or cream form, it's also known as cetyl-M.

CMO is advertised widely as a fast-acting cure for many forms of arthritis, but there is no scientific evidence at this time that these claims are true. The claims for CMO stem from a 1993 study showing that CMO injections prevented arthritis in rats. However, no evidence exists that the substance will work in humans. CMO's claims include lubricating joints, regulating the immune system, easing inflammation and reducing painful symptoms of many arthritis-related diseases.

One study on rats isn't reason enough to try a supplement that could be dangerous in people. Perhaps the most dangerous aspect of CMO is that some vendors advise people considering the supplement to stop taking methotrexate and corticosteroids first (explaining that these drugs could interfere with CMO's action). As we noted previously, this practice is very dangerous. You should *never* suddenly stop taking corticosteroids – this can be fatal. People with rheumatoid arthritis who stop taking their drugs to try CMO may develop further joint damage while they wait to see if the CMO works, and so may have more pain in the future.

Possible side effects: None known, but there is also no scientific evidence that CMO is safe to use.

Collagen

As we mentioned in the section on glucosamine and chondroitin, collagen is a common substance found in humans and animals. A protein, it is the chief component of cartilage, that cushioning, rubbery substance essential to healthy joint movement. Collagen is sold in supplement form as collagen hydrolysate or gelatin. There are many gelatin supplements on the market. Collagen supplements are made from cartilage of pigs, cows, oxen, chickens or sheep. It's available as a capsule, tablet or powder.

Collagen supplements supposedly relieve pain, inflammation and stiffness in people with various forms of arthritis. As collagen is a main component of cartilage, people take collagen on the assumption that it will repair deteriorated cartilage. But scientific evidence supporting these claims is controversial. A recent study found that pharmaceutical-grade collagen hydrolysate did not relieve pain in people with bone or joint disease any better than a placebo. But studies are still ongoing.

Possible side effects: Stomach upset and nausea. People with allergies to chicken or eggs should not take collagen supplements made from chickens.

Devil's Claw

Devil's claw, also known as grapple plant or wood spider, is made from a plant (*Harpagophytum procumbens*) found in Namibia and South Africa. The supplement contains the active ingredient harpagoside, which appears to reduce pain and inflammation in some joints.

It's sold in capsule, powdered root or tea form. Devil's claw may not just relieve pain and inflammation, but may also serve as a digestive aid or appetite stimulant, something that can appeal to people with chronic pain or fatigue who may have lost their appetite.

A recent clinical study on humans found that devil's claw relieved hip and knee osteoarthritis pain.

Possible side effects: Devil's claw may promote the secretion of stomach acid, so it should be avoided by anyone with gastric or duodenal ulcers, gastritis, or who is taking NSAIDs.

Dimethyl Sulfoxide (DMSO)

In the early 1960s, DMSO, a by-product of wood processing, was being hailed as a new therapy for all forms of arthritis. But studies of the substance were halted in the mid-'60s because high doses damaged the lens of the eye in animal studies. (No eye problems have been documented in human studies of DMSO.)

Today, DMSO is widely used in Russia and other countries for rheumatoid arthritis and osteoarthritis, but in the USA it has only one approved use – for a bladder condition called interstitial cystitis.

There is research that suggests DMSO can relieve pain and increase function for people with arthritis and that it may ease finger ulcers in scleroderma and relieve blood vessel constrictions in Raynaud's phenomenon. But the research is mixed. More studies are required to confirm DMSO's safety and effectiveness.

Possible side effects: Headache, dizziness, drowsiness, nausea, vomiting, diarrhoea, con-

stipation and loss of appetite. Topical DMSO can cause skin irritations or dermatitis.

Feverfew

Feverfew is made from the fresh or dried leaves of the feverfew plant (*Tanacetum parthenium*) commonly found in Europe. Available in capsule, tablet, fresh or dried leaf form, feverfew is used as a preventative for migraine headaches.

Animal studies show that feverfew may reduce inflammation, but human studies have found no benefit for people with arthritis.

Possible side effects: Stomach upset, diarrhoea, flatulence and vomiting. In chewable form, feverfew may cause mouth sores, irritation of the mouth, tongue or lips, and loss of taste. People with allergies to plants in the daisy family (chrysanthemum and marigolds) should avoid feverfew.

Flaxseed

Flaxseed, flaxseed oil or linseed oil is a very common food additive made from the seed of the flax plant (*Linum usitatissimum*). (Flax is also the source of the fabric linen.) Flaxseed is available as whole seeds, oil, capsules or as ground meal or flour. You might add it to foods or take it with water. Flaxseed or flaxseed oil supposedly relieves joint pain and stiffness and lubricates joints for easier movement.

Flaxseed contains alpha-linoleic acid, an omega-3 fatty acid. This is a term you may see frequently in the media. Omega-3 fatty acids are found in many food products, including some cold-water fish, such as salmon or tuna.

Omega-3 fatty acids have anti-inflammatory properties, one reason why doctors suggest adding these foods to your diet. However, the omega-3 fatty acids in flaxseed oil are not the same as those in oily fish, and do not have the same beneficial effects.

Possible side effects: Can act as a laxative and impair absorption of some medications.

Ginger

Ginger is a common spice added to many foods and used as an ingredient in baked goods and other cooked foods. Ginger supplements come from the dried or fresh root of the ginger plant, and are available in powder, extract, tincture, spice and oil form. They're widely available, and ginger root is sold in most supermarkets.

Ginger contains active ingredients that have analgesic and anti-inflammatory properties, and the root has long been used as an anti-nausea aid. One double-blind, clinical study of a highly purified ginger extract found that the supplement reduced knee osteoarthritis pain. However, the analgesic effects of ginger were small and inconsistent.

Possible side effects: Heartburn, diarrhoea and stomach discomfort. Ginger supplements may interfere with blood-pressure, blood-thinning, heart, diabetes or antacid medicines. People with gallstones should talk to their doctor before trying ginger supplements.

GLA

GLA, or gamma-linoleic acid, is an omega-6 fatty acid (a natural anti-inflammatory agent) found in various plant oils: evening primrose, black currant and borage. It is sold in capsule or oil form. People use GLA to reduce joint pain, swelling and stiffness, and to ease symptoms of some rheumatic diseases.

GLA may reduce inflammation in people with rheumatoid arthritis with few side effects.

Possible side effects: Evening primrose oil: indigestion, nausea, soft stools and headache. Borage seed oil: may exacerbate liver disease. Any type of GLA should be taken by mouth.

Green Tea

Much has been written about the health benefits of green tea, a widely consumed beverage throughout Asia and, increasingly, in the West. Green tea contains a substance that supposedly fights inflammation, and a concentrated version of this substance is available in capsule and tablet form. You can also buy and drink green tea in standard tea bags or loose leaves.

In some studies on animals, green tea has been found to have anti-inflammatory benefits, and laboratory studies also showed some promise that green tea reduces inflammation and slows the breakdown of cartilage. However, no human studies have shown any confirmed benefit for taking green tea if you have arthritis.

Possible side effects: Stomach upset, constipation. Green tea contains caffeine, so take this fact into account if you are sensitive to caffeine, pregnant or breastfeeding.

MSM

MSM is another supplement receiving wide attention from the media in recent years for its purported pain-relieving effects. MSM (short for methyl sulfonyl methane) is an organic sulfur compound found in many plants, animals and humans. This compound is necessary for the formation of connective tissue. In supplement form, it's available as a tablet, powder and topical ointment.

MSM supplements supposedly ease pain and inflammation. A few studies performed on animals support the notion that it eases inflammation. But more scientific, controlled studies are needed to be sure if MSM really works.

Possible side effects: None known at this time.

New Zealand Green-Lipped Mussel

Whilst you may dine on New Zealand green-lipped mussels at a fine restaurant, you may not know that a concentrated, freeze-dried, supplement version of the tasty shellfish is available as a complementary pain treatment. The mussels contain those inflammation-fighting omega-3 fatty acids as well as other substances believed to lessen painful inflammation.

Possible side effects: Diarrhoea, nausea, intestinal gas and liver problems. If you're allergic to shellfish, do not use.

SAM-e

S-adenosylmethionine, or SAM-e (pronounced 'sammy') for short, is a naturally occurring compound that is believed to improve joint mobility, relieve pain and ease depression. Although a number of European studies have shown that SAM-e relieves pain as effectively as several NSAIDs, in US studies SAM-e seemed to work for only mild pain.

Some studies have shown that SAM-e works as well as tricyclic antidepressants for depression – and with fewer side effects. One downside to SAM-e is its high cost. Any benefits last only as long as you take it.

Possible side effects: Flatulence, vomiting, diarrhoea, headache and nausea, but mostly these effects are seen when one has taken high doses of SAM-e. Should be avoided by people with bipolar disorder or Parkinson's disease. Could interact with antidepressants.

Sea Algae

One small study conducted recently suggested some pain-relief promise for a herbal supplement made from an extract of sea algae. Researchers process the algae and create an extract containing astaxanthin, a carotenoid, which is an antioxidant. (Astaxanthin causes the pink/orange colour in farmed salmon.)

Antioxidants are found in many foods and can help deactivate harmful particles, called free-radicals, produced by the body. But scientists still don't know how to best harness antioxidants or how much antioxidant-rich food or supplements to ingest to receive benefits. A healthy diet of foods rich in antioxidants may be superior to taking pills or supplements.

Sea algae extract is supposed to relieve pain associated with arthritis and carpal tunnel syndrome. Many more studies are needed to determine if sea algae extract works to help relieve pain.

Possible side effects: Shown to be safe when taken as directed.

Shark Cartilage

Cartilage is the flexible but firm substance that cushions many joints and helps us move more freely. Shark skeleton is mostly cartilage, one reason why the deep-sea predators move through the water with such ease and grace. Along with eating their meat and fins for dinner, people are using the fearsome fishes' cartilage as a nutritional supplement to ease pain and inflammation. It is ground and consumed as capsules, tablets, extract and powder.

Like other animals' cartilage, shark cartilage contains collagen, a substance believed by some to reduce pain and inflammation. It also contains calcium, a mineral known for its bone-building properties. Shark cartilage also contains chondroitin sulfate, which is used as a pain-and-inflammation-fighting supplement on its own (see p. 120). Some early studies on animals suggest that shark cartilage may be effective in reducing pain and inflammation.

Possible side effects: Dizziness, nausea, vomiting, stomach upset, constipation, stomach bloating, fatigue, low blood pressure, high blood sugar and high calcium levels.

Stinging Nettle

This common treatment is made from the stinging nettle plant's leaves and roots, and you consume it as a tea, tincture or extract, or use the leaves to apply directly to your skin. It may relieve pain, aches and inflammation.

Possible side effects: High in vitamin K, so may increase the risk of blood clots. Mild stomach upset.

Thunder God Vine

This dramatic-sounding supplement is an extract made from the leaf and root of an Asian plant. Extract of thunder god vine (scientific name *Tripterygium wilfordii Hook F*) supposedly relieves pain, inflammation and other symptoms in people with rheumatoid arthritis.

Few studies have been performed on humans to determine the effectiveness of thunder god vine. A recent small study by doctors at the US National Institutes of Health reported that their subjects, who had rheumatoid arthritis, experienced a reduction in symptoms compared with those who took a placebo supplement.

Yet this supplement may be dangerous for many people whom it's supposed to help. People taking immune system suppressing drugs such as prednisolone should not use extract of thunder god vine, as it could further suppress their immune systems. The leaves and flowers of the thunder god vine are poisonous, so use only extracts made from the plant's roots.

Possible side effects: Stomach upset, hair loss, heartburn, diarrhoea, skin reactions, loss of menstruation in women and temporary infertility in men.

KAVA KAVA: A POSSIBLY RISKY SUPPLEMENT

Kava kava is a herb, found in some herbal remedies. It is also sometimes found as an ingredient in food products.

Concerns have been raised recently about the safety of kava kava and its toxic effect on the liver. Of the 68 cases in the world suspected of being associated with the use of kava kava, three were in the UK.

The Committee on Safety of Medicines – the independent body that advises the Medicines Control Agency – has assessed this herbal ingredient and concluded that the risks outweigh any possible medical benefits. If you have been taking this herb, it would be wise to stop using it; there should not be any harm in stopping it suddenly.

Turmeric

Like ginger, turmeric is a commonly used spice added to many foods, such as curry. Made from a plant grown in India and Indonesia, it's a common ingredient in cuisines of those countries. Turmeric is related to the ginger family of plants. As a supplement, you may take it in capsule or powder form.

Turmeric is used to reduce pain and inflammation and to treat painful bursitis. It's a staple of Chinese and Indian Ayurvedic (traditional) medicine as an arthritis treatment and also as a digestive aid or body-cleansing agent. It may be used in combination with other common supplements. In fact, the only studies performed on turmeric have shown it may be effective in relieving arthritis-related pain when combined with boswellia, zinc, ginger or aswangandha (an Indian herbal treatment).

Possible side effects: Could cause stomach upset or thinning of blood when taken at high doses. If you have gallstones, do not use turmeric.

Willow Bark

Aspirin was first created from the bark of the willow, a beautiful tree common to many parts of the world. The active ingredient in the supplemental form of willow bark (or white willow) is salicin, which is very similar to salicylates, the active chemical in aspirin. People with arthritis, gout, ankylosing spondylitis, back problems and other painful arthritis-related diseases may use willow bark to ease muscle and joint aches and pains.

The drawback can be that it takes a great deal of willow bark to get enough of the pain-fighting ingredient, so it may be easier to take an aspirin. You might have to take willow bark tea or extract much longer to get the same benefit as aspirin pills. Willow bark is also available in a cream form for treating minor skin irritations.

Possible side effects: Similar to aspirin. Can increase the effect of blood thinners. Should not be used by children under 18 because of the risk of Reye's syndrome.

SUPPLEMENTS FOR FIBROMYALGIA

People with fibromyalgia experience a combination of symptoms, including muscle pain, aches, fatigue, sleeplessness and depression or anxiety. Because the root cause of fibromyalgia is not known, the disease can be hard to treat. Doctors usually respond by prescribing drugs to treat fibromyalgia's various symptoms. Supplements used by people with fibromyalgia often address sleep problems and mood-related symptoms.

If you have fibromyalgia, you may be curious about exploring natural supplements that might ease these symptoms as well. Below are several popular supplements for fibromyalgia symptoms. As we noted earlier in this chapter, talk to your doctor first if you wish to try one of these supplements. Some supplements may compound the effects of your prescribed drugs and cause problems. Note: SAM-e, described on p. 125, is also used by people with fibromyalgia to ease depression.

Ginseng

Many people throughout Asia use ginseng, a plant root, for various health benefits, including relief from stress and fatigue, a boost to the immune system, and an increase in physical stamina and cognitive function – all benefits that might appeal to a person with fibromyalgia. Ginseng's popularity has spread to the West, where many people use it as a 'pick-me-up'.

Sold as a fresh root or ground up in capsule, tablet, tea, tincture powder or tonic form, scientists do not know how or if ginseng really works. Few studies have been done and those that have show little or no benefit.

Possible side effects: Ginseng can increase the effects of corticosteroid medicines such as prednisolone. It can also cause insomnia, something people with fibromyalgia may be concerned about already, or act as a stimulant. People with heart conditions, hormone-sensitive conditions, diabetes, hypertension, low blood pressure or schizophrenia should avoid ginseng. Pregnant women, people who have had organ transplants or who are taking blood thinners, immunosuppressants or MAO inhibitors should avoid ginseng.

Grapeseed

Grapeseed extract or oil supplements come from the seeds of Asian grapes, and people can take it in tablet or capsule form. Grapeseed oil supposedly fights inflammation, improves circulation, and also relieves symptoms of fibromyalgia and chronic fatigue syndrome, a similar condition marked by severe, ongoing weariness.

Grapeseed oil is a powerful antioxidant, and it contains vitamin E, flavonoids and essential fatty acids, all substances known to be important to overall health. But no human studies have been performed, so its effectiveness is not proven.

Possible side effects: Can increase risk of bleeding, so do not use if you are taking drugs or supplements that have a blood-thinning effect.

Melatonin

Most people with fibromyalgia report trouble sleeping, and this lack of deep sleep may be one cause of their chronic pain. The body needs REM or deep sleep to rejuvenate its processes and restore energy for the coming day. People with fibromyalgia often don't get proper sleep, sparking a cycle of pain, fatigue and depression.

Melatonin supplement is derived from an animal version of a hormone found also in humans' pineal glands, located at the base of the brain. It comes in capsule, tablet, liquid, lozenge or tea form.

Melatonin is a powerful antioxidant, and it may regulate the human sleep cycle to reduce insomnia or the restless, disturbed sleep common in fibromyalgia. Taking aspirin and other NSAIDs may lower the body's natural melatonin levels. Studies suggest that melatonin may boost the immune system and bone growth, but no valid clinical studies prove its effectiveness as a sleep aid. Melatonin should not be used for longer than two weeks.

Possible side effects: May interact with heart or depression medicines and immunosuppressants. Don't mix with alcohol as it could dangerously intensify the effect, and do not take along with similar sleep-promoting supplements such as valerian. Do not use if you have rheumatoid arthritis or lupus.

St John's Wort

This popular supplement is an extract of a wild plant with yellow flowers, St John's wort, which grows in North America and Europe. It's sold in powder, liquid, tablet, capsule or tea form.

People take St John's wort as an antidepressant and to reduce muscle pain common in fibromyalgia. Researchers believe the plant contains active ingredients that boost levels of serotonin, a brain chemical that may be linked to the pain, sensitivity and sleep problems of fibromyalgia. People need to take St John's wort for up to a month before seeing its benefits, and they may experience withdrawal symptoms if they suddenly stop taking the supplement.

St John's wort may relieve mild to moderate, but not severe, depression. You should only take St John's wort with your doctor's approval, as it can interact with some medications. St John's wort should not be taken by people taking antidepressants.

Possible side effects: Sensitivity to sunlight, dizziness, insomnia, fatigue, anxiety, stomach upset and dry mouth.

Valerian Root

A popular herbal sleep aid, valerian root is used widely in Europe to help sleeplessness and to ease muscle and joint pain. Valerian, a pungent, ground plant root, is sold in capsule, tablet, extract or tea form. Valerian teas are very strong-tasting and may be unpalatable to some people.

Valerian is a mild sedative and aids sleep. Clinical studies suggest it is an effective insomnia treatment, but no studies have proven its effectiveness for pain relief. Do not take with alcohol or other sedatives, as it might intensify the effects.

Possible side effects: Headache, insomnia and excitability. Do not use for longer than four weeks.

VITAMINS, MINERALS AND DIETARY CHANGES

Many doctors and health-care professionals suggest a diet rich in vitamins, minerals and nutrients for good health. Can a higher intake of certain vitamins and minerals – or even a change in what foods you eat – cause or lessen your pain? It's not likely that popping a particular vitamin pill each day will help to relieve pain, but research does show the power of certain nutrients to control painful diseases such as arthritis, osteoporosis and more.

In addition, some people subscribe to a theory that particular diets will help control pain and inflammation. There is not enough evidence to support these theories, but there are safe, healthy ways to test whether certain foods trigger or worsen your pain.

One of the few conditions clearly linked to diet is gout. People with gout should follow a diet that eliminates or greatly reduces the consumption of foods high in purines. In general, doctors and health experts recommend a varied diet, rich in fresh fruit and vegetables, vitamins, minerals and nutrients, and low in fatty or processed foods. If you do have a chronic pain condition, you may wish to include foods rich in particular nutrients, such as omega-3 fatty acids (common in oily fish) that can reduce inflammation, or foods rich in antioxidants, nutrients that help fight the effects of *free radicals,* molecules in the environment that play a role in the ageing and disease processes.

Gout and Diet

Gout, which usually results from a high level of uric acid in the blood, is one of the few chronic pain conditions that clearly can be helped by cutting back on certain foods. However, because drugs such as allopurinol and probenecid work so well to control painful gout attacks, some people with gout may rely on their drugs to control the pain rather than avoiding what may have caused the condition in the first place: their purine-rich diets.

People with gout can lower uric acid levels in their blood by avoiding foods high in purines. These include organ meats (e.g. liver, kidneys), pâté, wild or farmed game, fish roe, meat extracts (e.g. Bovril, Vegemite), scallops, mackerel, herring, trout, crayfish, lobster, small fish eaten whole or processed (e.g. anchovies, whitebait, anchovy paste). Foods that can be eaten in moderation include red meat, poultry, dried beans or peas, brassicas, spinach, asparagus, avocado, mushrooms.

There are a few other steps to reduce the chances of a gout attack:

- **Limit alcoholic beverages** (especially beer), as they may increase uric acid levels in the blood.

- **Don't fast**, as this could increase uric acid levels in the blood and trigger an attack.

- **Control your weight**, but reduce excess weight gradually.

- **Drink plenty of water** – at least two litres daily – so your kidneys can work properly and excrete uric acid.

Is Food a Pain Trigger?

Could certain foods be pain triggers or disease fighters? Experts have not yet confirmed this to be true, but more information is being discovered about the links between nutrition and disease.

One chronic pain condition triggered by certain foods is headaches, such as migraine headaches. People with chronic headaches should consider avoiding potential trigger foods, including chocolate, red wine or red wine vinegars, the seasoning monosodium glutamate, aged cheeses, processed meats, and foods or beverages containing caffeine.

Only about 2 per cent of the population suffers from true food allergies, where even a tiny amount of a certain food elicits a serious allergic response. But many people may be sensitive to certain foods. If they have a chronic pain condition, eating certain foods could make them feel worse. If a person has a chronic inflammatory condition, a diet high in foods such as saturated animal fats and many vegetable oils might contribute to joint and tissue inflammation that causes serious pain.

In the past, many 'arthritis diets' have circulated, perpetuated further by the creation of the Internet. These diets claim to cure arthritis or greatly reduce pain simply by eliminating certain foods. These claims are unproven. Unlike the headache triggers, no particular food has been proven to trigger joint pain, arthritis or inflammation.

However, two facts about diet and arthritis are true. One, if you are overweight, you increase your risk of developing osteoarthritis or making any type of arthritis worse. Excess weight puts additional strain on joints, and if your joints are damaged or weakened due to arthritis, they don't need extra strain. Two, there are some reports that support the idea that certain nutrients (including particular oils, vegetables and animal products) may either help or worsen joint pain. Some doctors might suggest you use more 'good' oils such as olive, rapeseed or flaxseed, and less 'bad' oils, such as corn or safflower, in your diet. Oils rich in omega-6 fatty acids may contribute to inflammation, whilst oils rich in omega-3 fatty acids (found in oily fish, flaxseed oil and other foods) may be beneficial to people with inflammation.

Many Internet sites and magazine stories promote the idea of adopting extreme diets as a way to fight disease. Switching from your balanced diet to a radically different diet lacking whole food groups may do more harm than good, depriving you of important nutrients. Some diets promote certain combinations of foods as magic 'cures' for arthritis or chronic pain, but there is no evidence to support such claims.

At present, theories linking foods to pain or

inflammation are mostly just that: theories. Only hearsay and uncontrolled studies provide any basis for these theories. Because many people with chronic pain have serious illnesses that vary in severity over time, it's difficult to determine what may cause their flares.

Some research does support the link between food and pain. Red meat and many vegetable oils, including corn, sunflower and safflower oils contain omega-6 fatty acids, which break down into arachidonic acid in the body. This one of the building blocks for prostaglandins and leukotrienes that can cause pain and inflammation. It is possible to eat a diet lower in some of these foods by choosing poultry, fish or vegetarian meals and using olive or rapeseed oils for cooking. You might improve your heart's health and your weight in the process. Another theory is the 'leaky gut' syndrome. This theory contends that some diseases, including arthritis, fibromyalgia, Crohn's disease and others, may cause the intestines to become leaky or porous, allowing tiny molecules from foods or bacteria to slip through to the rest of the body. The theory is that the leaks lead to inflammation, pain and exacerbated immune system problems. There is no scientific evidence to support this theory.

How can you tell if a certain food may be causing or worsening your pain? Keep a food diary. Take note of everything you eat for at least one week. Make sure you note the various ingredients of your foods. Read the labels of different products you use and ask questions about the foods you eat in restaurants. Take note of foods, seasonings or additives used in various dishes, including sauces. Write down what alcoholic beverages you consume and how much. Make sure you note the date and time when you ate or drank these items.

Also take note of when you experienced pain. Did a painful flare occur just after eating a particular meal? What did that meal contain? Watch for times when you ate other meals containing those ingredients. If you detect a pattern, try eliminating that one ingredient from your diet for a week or two. See if your pain subsides. On the flip side, you might try adding certain foods, such as the 'good' oils listed earlier (see p. 131), in moderate amounts and keeping track of any beneficial changes you detect over time.

What foods are the most commonly reported triggers of pain? Although they do not apply to every person experiencing pain or inflammation, below is a short list:

Dairy foods. Some people believe that dairy foods can worsen inflammatory forms of arthritis. Whilst this is not proven, you can try a dairy-free diet, but it is important to maintain healthy levels of calcium with soy, vegetables and other foods, or calcium supplements. Get the help of a registered dietitian.

Nightshade vegetables. Some people believe that eating vegetables in the *Solanaceae* or nightshade family leads to joint inflammation. These foods include tomatoes, potatoes, aubergines and peppers. Horticulturist Norman F. Childers, PhD, first proposed this theory; his diverticulitis (a painful inflammation of part of the intestines) flared after he ate nightshade vegetables. However, many doctors believe that the nightshade theory is speculative at best and may be completely wrong.

Food additives or seasonings. Additives or seasonings such as monosodium glutamate (MSG), nitrates or salt may cause unpleasant or painful reactions in some people. These additives are common in processed or packaged foods, cured meats such as bacon or luncheon meat, and meals prepared in restaurants.

Other purported pain triggers. Red meat, pork, eggs, peanuts, coffee, wheat, aspartame and corn have all been mentioned as possible triggers of pain. There is no scientific evidence to prove that these foods do lead to flares of pain. If you believe eating these foods has contributed to flares of your pain, talk to your doctor before eliminating anything from your diet or assuming you have an 'allergy' – a sensitivity – to these foods.

Diets that eliminate whole groups of foods – such as all carbohydrates, vegetables, fruits, fats or proteins – are not healthy eating plans. It's important to eat a diet that is balanced, so you receive all the nutrients your body needs to run properly. For example, if you choose a vegetarian diet in an effort to lose weight or improve your health, you need to compensate for the eliminated meat protein with plant-based proteins, such as tofu or beans.

Another pain-fighting practice that could be dangerous to your health is fasting, or abstaining from food for a period of time. Some fasts allow the person to only drink water or fruit juice for several days. The theory behind fasting as a therapy is that the fast cleanses the body of toxins or any foods that may have caused pain. After the fast, the person then starts adding one food at a time until they determine what foods may cause pain.

It is not recommended that you fast for any period of time if you have a chronic illness or chronic pain. This is especially so if you are taking medications for pain. Don't fast unless your doctor specifically advises you to abstain from food (such as if you are having surgery or undergoing a certain test). Fasting can lead to weakness, dizziness, dehydration and other problems. Fasting can trigger attacks in people with gout.

What about foods you might add to your diet to increase joint health or decrease pain? Could certain vitamin or nutrient supplements help as well? Striking the right balance of oils and omega fatty acids in your diet may help fight inflammation. Rapeseed and olive oils also have a better balance of good fatty acids than corn, sunflower or safflower oil, which are high in omega-6 fatty acids and can lead to inflammation. Using small amounts of rapeseed and olive oil in your food preparation can also encourage better heart health.

Some people take fish oil supplements instead of eating a lot of fish meals to get the health benefits of the omega-3 fatty acids. They can also add flaxseed to their foods. (Flaxseed can act as a laxative; use it with this in mind.) Gamma-linoleic acid (GLA), usually taken in supplement form as borage oil, evening primrose oil or black currant seed oil, can also help fight painful inflammation. GLA can aid in the body's production of series 1-prostaglandins, which can fight inflammation.

Vitamins and Minerals

The idea of 'taking your vitamins' suggests that getting the right nutrients, whether through a balanced diet or a supplement, can boost good health. Some people believe that doses of certain vitamins can prevent or treat illness as well. Research is beginning to prove them right in certain cases, although using vitamins in the same way we use drugs is not likely to offer pain relief.

What is a vitamin? Vitamins are natural organic substances necessary for normal metabolism. The word 'vitamin' was first used by Polish biochemist Casimir Funk in the early 20th century. Dr Funk studied chickens that developed a nerve inflammation, or neuritis. He discovered that the cause of the inflammation was a lack of a certain nutrient in the chickens' diet. Dr Funk named the nutrient a 'vitamine,' combining the Latin term *vita,* or life, with the word *amine,* referring to chemical compounds that contain nitrogen (we now know vitamins don't have to contain nitrogen). Later, newly discovered vitamins were identified with letters of the alphabet: A, B, C, D, E, K and so on.

Minerals are inorganic substances that come from the earth. Certain minerals, such as iron, selenium, zinc and calcium, are necessary for the body's growth and the normal functioning of many body processes. When we have a deficiency of essential minerals, physical sickness can result. Many multivitamin supplements contain a mixture of vitamins and minerals that are designed to make up for any deficiencies in your dietary intake of these nutrients. However, it is always preferable to get your vitamins and minerals from a healthy, varied diet rather than from a pill. Your doctor may determine that you need additional supplements of certain vitamins or minerals for disease prevention or good health.

Can vitamin or mineral supplements ease pain? It's unlikely, but with a doctor's supervision, these supplements can be part of an overall disease-prevention and pain-management plan. Some vitamins and minerals help prevent *cell oxidation.* Oxidation is a natural process in which a substance combines with oxygen, present in the atmosphere. When metal rusts, the substance of the metal is combining with the air around it, and the oxidation results in rust. Whilst the process of cells oxidizing isn't the same as your body rusting from within, it is true that cells can break down in the oxidation process. Certain vitamins and other nutrients combat this process by working as antioxidants. Antioxidants can help prevent cell breakdown that might lead to serious, painful diseases such as arthritis or cancer.

Although you can take multivitamin supplements or vitamin and mineral pills that contain antioxidants, it's best to get most of your nutrients from the foods you eat. When you eat a varied diet of fresh foods, you are more likely to get all the vitamins you need, along with fibre, iron and other important nutrients. Multivitamin supplements can complement a healthy diet, but shouldn't replace it. Good food sources of these nutrients include:

- **Beta-carotene:** Carrots, sweet potatoes and leafy green vegetables

- **Vitamin A:** Liver, carrots and other vegetables and dairy produce

- **Vitamin C:** Citrus fruits, berries, tomatoes, and most vegetables

- **Vitamin E:** Nuts, leafy green vegetables, wheat germ, liver and sweet potatoes

- **Selenium:** Seafood, organ meats, and some grains and seeds, especially Brazil nuts

- **Vitamin B:** Found in many foods

- **Vitamin K:** Green vegetables, cheese, oats; can also be made in the gut

Vitamin D is another important nutrient that may help people with chronic pain conditions, including osteoarthritis. Vitamin D is produced by the body when exposed to sunlight, and is also found in dairy products. Low levels of vitamin D have been found in people with osteoarthritis. This may be because some people with chronic pain do not get outdoors regularly, especially if their pain keeps them in bed or on the sofa. They may get even less sunlight exposure during cold, winter months when the weather can be bad and there are fewer hours of daylight. Supplements of the vitamin and new, safe sunlight lamps may be helpful.

Any vitamin or mineral deficiency can cause disease; for example, scurvy is due to vitamin C deficiency. But, today, such diseases caused by vitamin deficiency are very rare. However, low levels of essential vitamins and minerals in your diet could be a contributing factor to the development of more complex diseases such as arthritis, osteoporosis, heart disease and cancer.

Calcium and **iron** are two essential minerals. Calcium helps you build strong bones. Good sources of calcium include milk or dairy products, fortified cereals or juices, leafy green vegetables and tinned sardines or salmon with bones. Iron is essential for the prevention of anaemia, a lower than normal count of red blood cells. People with anaemia can experience fatigue and tire easily.

Over the years, research has been conducted about the possible links between a lack of certain vitamins and various health problems. For example, a person who does not get enough calcium in their diet is at a higher risk for developing osteoporosis. People with osteoarthritis often have lower levels of vitamins C and D in their bodies.

The question that follows is: Can taking extra amounts of certain vitamins prevent or relieve painful conditions? Most doctors don't recommend taking high doses of vitamins, as many become toxic at high concentrations. Overuse of vitamin or mineral supplements, even ones you may consider healthy, could lead to other health problems. So it's important to take vitamins or minerals only after clearing it with your doctor.

There is a view that aspirin and NSAIDs can cause vitamins and other supplements to break down more quickly and easily, decreasing their effectiveness. So you might like to take your vitamin or other supplements two to three hours before or after you take your NSAID.

It's also important for people with any chronic illness or chronic pain condition to have a nutritious diet and take vitamin supplements if necessary. Some medications used by people with chronic illness (who may take these drugs over a long period of time) may lower the amount of certain nutrients in their body. For example, methotrexate, a drug taken by many people with rheumatoid arthritis, severe asthma and other diseases, may lower levels of folic acid, an important nutrient, in the body. Folic acid – which is found in many enriched breakfast cereals –

helps prevent birth defects, but it also plays a key role in the production of SAM-e (see p. 125) in the body, which helps maintain healthy cartilage. Folic acid supplements may lower the severity or frequency of the serious side effects of methotrexate, so there is an added benefit to taking this supplement while on methotrexate.

Many people with chronic illness have low levels of certain nutrients in their blood, and they may not get enough exercise or eat a proper diet because of fatigue, depression, side effects of medications or constant pain. So nutritional supplements may be helpful.

The link between vitamins and minerals and disease is complex. It's important not to try to treat yourself with nutritional supplements, but instead to rely on the advice of your doctor. Ask your doctor if you should take a multivitamin supplement or if you need concentrated amounts of a particular vitamin or mineral. The best approach is a broad one, with a healthy diet, regular exercise and proper medications.

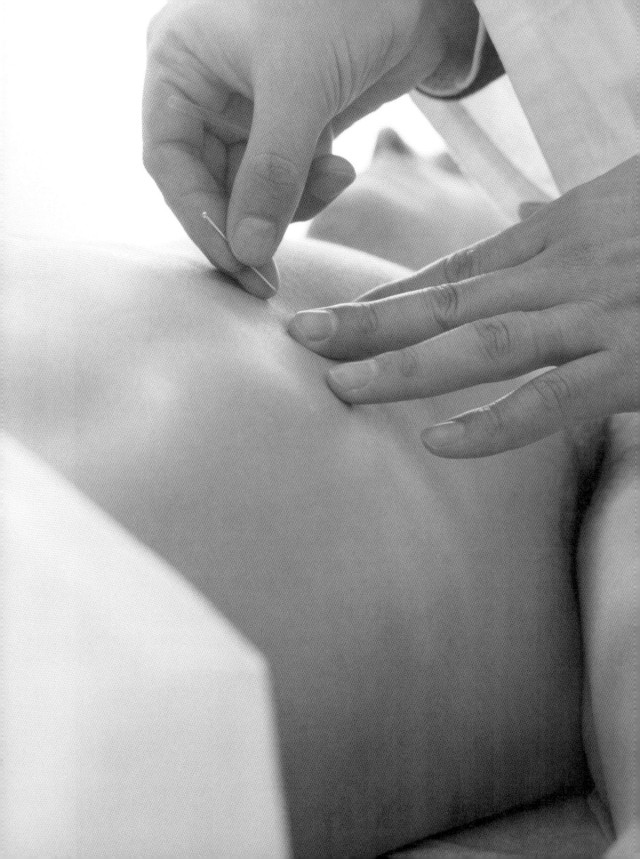

Massage, Manipulation and Other Therapies

8

CHAPTER 8: MASSAGE, MANIPULATION AND OTHER THERAPIES

Most complementary therapies for pain relief don't involve taking herbs or nutritional supplements. There are many other philosophies of healing, as well as treatments performed by practitioners of these philosophies, that are increasing in popularity for people with chronic pain.

Some of these treatments rise from ancient healing traditions in China or India. Others stem from relatively recent health philosophies. No matter how old or new these complementary treatments are, they tend to spark controversy, as well as debate among doctors and their patients.

No matter what therapy you try, it's important to find out if the practitioner is a member of the relevant professional society (see the Resources section) and has the proper training to perform the procedures. Never allow a practitioner who is not properly licensed to perform any type of manipulation or treatment on your body. You should agree on fees and terms beforehand so you will know what charges you will owe for these services.

Consult your GP also so he knows what therapies you are exploring. In some cases, your doctor can refer you to reputable, qualified practitioners of various therapies. Some doctors also perform these therapies as part of their integrative practice. In addition, some physiotherapists, occupational thera-

pists or other health-care professionals may offer some of these services.

ACUPUNCTURE AND ACUPRESSURE

Acupuncture is an ancient, Asian healing technique that has gained popularity in the West over the past few decades. Mainstream medical institutions now take acupuncture seriously and are studying the therapy to determine why and how well it works. Many UK national charities and research organizations have funded research on acupuncture to explore its effectiveness.

Acupuncture is part of *Chinese medicine.* Chinese medicine, which may also involve herbs, massage, meditation techniques or exercises, developed over thousands of years in China, but has gained new popularity in the West in recent years. One of the main reasons people seek acupuncture treatment is to relieve chronic pain, especially back pain, arthritis or fibromyalgia. Currently, a number of scientific studies are being conducted to research the effectiveness and safety of acupuncture treatment specifically for osteoarthritis and other diseases involving chronic pain.

Acupuncture involves a trained professional puncturing the skin with very thin needles at any of 300 specific sites on the body. These points lie along energy pathways called *meridians.* Devotees of acupuncture believe that the placement of needles at these points will increase the energy flow (called qi; pronounced *chee*) along the meridians. Qi is, in traditional Chinese belief, essential to healthy balance in the body, known as yin and yang. *Acupressure* is another form of this treatment, but one involving hand pressure rather than needle punctures.

Acupuncture supposedly boosts the body's natural ability to heal itself and relieve pain.

Studies about acupuncture have found some merit to these claims. They find that some people have higher levels of endorphins, those natural pain-fighting chemicals the body produces, in their cerebrospinal fluid after acupuncture.

Scientists do not yet understand why pricking the skin at these particular points causes the endorphin boost, or why acupuncturists place their needles in one part of the body to get pain relief in another part. Acupuncture may stimulate the flow of electromagnetic signals through the body along the meridians, helping endorphins flow. Acupuncture may also activate the release of the central nervous system's natural opiates (similar to the chemicals in opiate drugs), which relieve pain. Or it may aid in the release of certain neurotransmitters, body chemicals that play a role in how the brain relays pain messages, and *neurohormones*, brain chemicals that can affect the function of the body's organs.

More scientific studies are necessary if acupuncture is to be established as a pain-relief treatment, but the procedure may well provide relief from many painful conditions, including headache, tennis elbow, fibromyalgia, myofascial pain, osteoarthritis, low back pain, carpal tunnel syndrome and more. Most doctors who support the use of acupuncture believe it should be used as a complement to regular medical treatment of chronic pain. Many countries have licensing boards that license acupuncturists and other individuals who practise 'healing arts' to perform treatments. In the UK, consult the British Acupuncture Council (see the Resources section for their details).

What Happens During Acupuncture? During an acupuncture session, the practitioner (known as an acupuncturist) will take a medical history and examine you (particularly your pulses and your tongue) to help him make a traditional Chinese medicine diagnosis. He will then select a number of points on your body to use in your treatment. Using a new sterile needle each time, the acupuncturist will insert the needles and leave them there while you lie on a table for about 20 minutes. He may rotate the needles during this time – a practice thought to achieve greater effect. (In acupressure, he applies pressure, not needles, to these points.) Some acupuncturists also use electrical stimulation of the needles to boost the procedure's effects, a procedure known as *electroacupuncture*. Others use dried herbs as part of their treatment of the patient, a practice called *moxibustion.*

The acupuncturist will then remove the needles and will probably ask you to rest some more before rising from the table. Reactions to the procedure vary widely from person to person. You may feel light-headed or drowsy, so you should not drive yourself home from your first session. Usually, repeated treatments are needed for relief of chronic pain.

To find an acupuncturist in your area, first ask your doctor for a referral. If he cannot give you any information, consult the British Acupuncture Council, the national body that certifies acupuncturists. (See the Resources section for contact details.)

Acupressure. Acupressure is a massage-like technique where the practitioner presses on particular points of the body in an attempt to relieve pain that may occur in other areas of the body. According to the theory behind the therapy, these acupoints occur on energy pathways, or meridians, as in acupuncture, and the therapy is designed to restore proper energy flow and balance to relieve pain.

MANIPULATION THERAPIES

One popular treatment for pain relief, particularly of chronic neck and back pain or post-injury pain, is *manipulation therapy,* or manual adjustment of the spine or the limbs in order to restore proper alignment or promote the body's natural healing ability. Many different health-care professionals perform manipulation therapy, and the therapy they offer may vary slightly from discipline to discipline. Chiropractors are probably the most common practitioners of this therapy, but osteopaths, physiotherapists and even some doctors may also perform it.

Chiropractic and Osteopathy

Chiropractic is a system that holds that pain and many other health problems, including minor and serious diseases, occur because the body's spine is out of alignment. Chiropractors perform regular adjustments to the spine, or *spinal manipulations,* in order to restore the spine to its optimal position. According to the philosophy of chiropractic, a well-adjusted spine allows the body to perform its natural defences of pain and disease at optimal levels.

Whilst there is dispute among scientists as to the validity of the theory of chiropractic, many people seek chiropractors and other health-care professionals for periodic or regular spinal manipulation as a therapy for pain. Whether or not the therapy works, or whether or not the overall philosophy behind it is valid, is a matter of opinion at this point.

Chiropractic began in 1895 in Iowa, when a lay healer named David Daniel Palmer formed the basic theory of what was then called vertebral subluxations. His treatment philosophy spread.

In the UK, chiropractors are registered with the General Chiropractic Council, the statutory body for regulating the profession. Over 50 per cent of chiropractors are represented by the British Chiropractic Association (BCA); they will have undergone a four-year full-time internationally accredited degree course. Chiropractors cannot prescribe drugs or perform surgery, but they do consult with patients and perform manipulation and other treatments.

Osteopathy was founded in the 19th century, by a US Civil War surgeon named Andrew Still, who was disillusioned by the failures of the mainstream medicine of his time. He devised his own theory that the body's musculoskeletal system was key to good health and the body's ability to defend itself against disease and to heal itself following injury.

Osteopathy uses many of the same practices and follows many of the same principles as traditional or allopathic medicine. In the examination room, osteopathic treatment may be quite similar to examinations by a doctor. However, osteopaths may focus more on general health and wellness practices, as well as addressing the home and work environment of the patient.

As osteopathic medicine is based on the idea that the musculoskeletal system is at the root of many diseases and pain conditions, osteopaths receive additional training in treating the musculoskeletal system. Their treatment may include *osteopathic manipulative treatment,* using their hands on the body of the patient in an effort to diagnose disease, damage to tissues and more. Treatment may also include manipulation, where the osteopath uses his hands more forcefully to correct problems in the musculoskeletal system.

What Happens During Manipulation Therapy? Manipulation therapy usually follows a consultation with the practitioner. He may determine your range of motion (the amount of flexibility you have in certain joints), muscle tone or strength, reflexes and more. Then, the practitioner might perform the manipulation therapy, along with prescribing treatments and suggestions, such as exercise or dietary changes.

Spinal manipulation involves the practitioner using either his hands or a small pushing instrument to press on the spine, back and neck or, sometimes, the limbs. The manipulation often looks as if they are pushing or stretching your neck and back into alignment, while you lie on your stomach on a padded table. You may hear a crack or pop, but this is simply air being released from the moving vertebrae. The practitioner may get you to rest for a few moments after the manipulation.

Study results and professional opinions are mixed on the benefit of spinal manipulation therapy for people with chronic pain. You may have to rely on your own judgement as to whether this therapy is worth trying. If you try spinal manipulation therapy and do not see some relief after three or four sessions, it probably isn't going to work. You may receive some pain relief from the manipulations, but if you don't see improvement, try massage, water therapy, exercise or other techniques instead.

Be wary of any practitioner who claims that continual manipulations throughout your lifetime are necessary to achieving pain relief and good health; there is no evidence to support this claim. Also, be wary of any practitioner who suggests that you discontinue any other medical treatment or seeing your medical doctors for care.

Although it's likely that spinal manipulation is safe, people with inflammatory arthritis or osteoporosis should use caution because manipulation might damage weakened joints or bones. Fracture of bones can occur. It's essential to inform your chiropractor, osteopath, physiotherapist or any other spinal manipulation practitioner about your health conditions. Don't just say, 'I'm in pain.' Practitioners need to know any possible health problems you may have in order to perform manipulation properly. If manipulation causes pain, stop the treatment and inform the practitioner.

Your doctor should be able to refer you to a qualified practitioner of manipulation therapy in your area. Chiropractors and osteopaths are required by law to be registered with the relevant regulatory body: the General Chiropractic Council and the General Osteopathic Council Association.

Craniosacral Therapy

A similar form of manipulation therapy, although one less widely practised, is *craniosacral therapy*. This therapy aims to balance the fluids in what practitioners term the craniosacral system – the fluids that run down your spinal cord from the brain to the base of the spine. Practitioners and devotees believe an imbalance in this fluid can cause various health problems, including pain.

In craniosacral therapy, the practitioner stands behind you while you lie on a comfortable table, and gently holds your head in his hands while applying soft pressure to various points on the back of the neck. He may also apply gentle pressure to points at the base of the spine. Experts are very divided on the validity or usefulness of this procedure. Some people find it beneficial or relaxing.

Some chiropractors and osteopaths perform *cranial manipulation*, in which they apply gentle pressure to the skull in certain areas in order to relieve pain. They use the heels of their hands and press on particular points of the skull. Some professionals use this technique to relieve chronic neck and back pain, ear pain, and even *tinnitus* (a chronic ringing or buzzing in the ears). Some of these practitioners believe that the cranial manipulation doesn't relieve the pain, but corrects misalignment of the skull's bones (which actually don't move) so the body's natural defence system can work more effectively.

MASSAGE

Massage is a common procedure used by many people who are not in chronic pain but enjoy the soothing action of massage for stress relief or improvement in flexibility. But many people use massage for pain relief, and studies show that this is an effective, safe therapy when administered by a qualified professional. Massage therapists are plentiful and located in almost every area, and their fees should be affordable.

'Massage' is a common term and there are several different types of massage. In a nutshell, massage is the manual manipulation and kneading of soft tissues, particularly muscles. Massage's benefits include improved blood circulation, relaxation of tense muscles, improved range of motion and increased endorphin levels – all of which may benefit people with chronic pain. Massage may enable you to feel more flexible and relaxed, so you sleep better and are more able to exercise regularly to maintain good health.

Below is a rundown of the different types of massage therapy. Ask your doctor or physiotherapist to suggest what type of massage is appropriate for your type of pain.

Swedish massage. This is the most common form of massage, and the form most people think of when they hear 'massage'. Swedish massage therapists knead the top layers of muscles of the body, often applying lotion or oil to ease their hand movements. Swedish massage usually lasts between 30 minutes and an hour. Some sessions are relaxing and others involve harder, more vigorous pressing designed to loosen tense muscles.

Deep tissue massage. This type of massage therapy involves a deeper, harder pressing by the therapist in order to release tension in the deepest layers of soft tissue. Therapists might use their fingers, elbows or thumbs to press between layers of muscles and get to the sources of pain or tension. Some people may experience soreness after the first few sessions, but later may find relief of nagging pain, such as low back pain or arthritis.

Trigger point therapy or neuromuscular massage. Trigger points are painful or tense points in the body that may be triggering pain elsewhere. In order to release the muscle tension that may be causing pain, practitioners use their fingers to press deeply into the body and massage those points. Some people with fibromyalgia find this therapy useful for temporary pain relief, but it can be a painful experience for others.

Myofascial release massage. Myofascial pain is centred in the fascia – the fibrous, thin connective tissues beneath the skin, sheathing your muscles. In this massage therapy, practitioners gently massage and stretch the fascia in order to release tension in these structures. Typically, myofascial release therapy sessions last about 30 minutes, and don't use oil as in Swedish massage. People with myofascial pain, as well as fibromyalgia and pain caused by tension or stress, may find relief with this therapy.

Oriental massage techniques. As we discussed on p. 140, many Oriental medicine practitioners perform techniques designed to restore the flow of qi in the body. *Shiatsu* massage is a Japanese technique that is gaining popularity in the West and is widely available at spas and health clubs where massage is offered. It's similar to acupressure because it aims to improve the flow of energy along the meridians. Sessions may take place on a table or a mat on the floor, and include stretching techniques as well.

A less widely practised Oriental massage technique is *tuina,* a Chinese therapy that includes massaging the body's pressure points.

Rolfing. Rolfing (named for its inventor, Ida Rolf) involves a technique very similar to deep tissue massage, and the idea is that tightness in the fascia may be causing pain. Rolfing aims to release muscles and other soft tissues from the fascia so that the body can restore its natural healing ability, aiming more at body maintenance than treating disease. Usually, Rolfing therapy takes place in ten one-hour sessions held about a week apart.

Hellerwork is a similar, massage-based practice that also involves exercises and teaching the person better posture and movement techniques in order to prevent pain.

Skinrolling technique. Some people with fibromyalgia find pain relief from this type of massage. Skinrolling involves a therapist picking up a roll of the person's skin and moving it carefully back and forth across the fascia, the fibrous tissues underneath. This technique aims to break the connections between the tissue and the nerve endings under them that are communicating the pain messages. Skinrolling can be painful at first, so therapists may use a mild anaesthetic before the treatment. Some people have reported long-lasting relief from fibromyalgia pain after skinrolling, but others find the technique itself too painful.

Spray and stretch technique. This kind of massage is used by people with fibromyalgia and also by people experiencing chronic back pain. Experts are divided as to its validity. Spray and stretch is usually performed by a physiotherapist rather than a massage therapist. The doctor or therapist sprays the skin over the painful area with a cooling anaesthetic, such as ethyl chloride, and then gently kneads the tense, painful muscles.

With any type of massage therapy, you should feel some relief after the session or at least in a few days. Most people who rely on massage therapy for pain relief schedule appointments regularly, as often as their doctor or physiotherapist might suggest.

To find a qualified therapist, ask your doctor for a referral, or consult a physiotherapy clinic or pain clinic in your area. If you use the services of a spa, make sure you check the credentials of the practitioners – they should be trained professionals. Be wary of so-called 'massage parlours' or 'health spas', which may offer cheaply priced massages performed by untrained people.

You can also perform your own massage to certain areas of the body that may be painful, such as wrists, arms, legs, feet, neck or shoulders. It may be difficult for you to reach your own back, but you may be able to massage your own lower back. Massage devices are available at many shops. These devices can help you massage sore joints or muscles, and some can apply soothing heat as well.

Reflexology

Somewhat similar to massage but more focused on a specific area of the body, *reflexology* is a pain-relief technique that is more akin to acupressure than traditional Swedish, full-body massage.

Reflexology practitioners believe that the hands, feet and ears have particular pressure points that correlate to different areas of the body or organs. When they apply pressure to these points, the correlating body part that is painful will experience pain relief. For example, pressing on the heel might aid pain in the sciatic nerve, which is located in the back. Whether or not this theory is valid – and there are few studies to suggest that it is – some people find the treatment soothing and relaxing. This may be due to the placebo effect because they believe that the treatment will ease their pain.

OTHER PAIN-RELIEF THERAPIES

There are numerous pain-relief therapies that either fall outside the standard medical treatment spectrum or are somewhat experimental. Many of these therapies are performed or prescribed by doctors and other mainstream health-care professionals, such as physiotherapists. Before trying any of these therapies, talk to your doctor and, if you have private health insurance, check the policy for coverage.

TENS

Earlier in the book, we discussed implants that release electrical stimulation of nerves in order to relieve pain. (See p. 106.) Another type of electricity-based therapy is TENS, or transcutaneous electrical nerve stimulation. TENS uses electrical stimulation to the nerves to block pain signals from getting to the brain. Many doctors now suggest that their patients try this pain treatment, especially people with back pain, arthritis, fibromyalgia or nerve-related pain. You can administer TENS yourself.

TENS is not painful and requires no needles, surgery or drugs, so it's gaining in popularity as a treatment for chronic pain. Usually, TENS helps people with pain concentrated in a particular area of the body, rather than all-over pain.

What Happens During TENS? Your doctor or another practitioner will place small electrodes on your skin in the area where you are experiencing pain. The electrodes are connected to a small, battery-operated box that releases low-level electricity. When the box passes a current, you feel a tingling sensation. If successful, TENS provides temporary pain relief.

TENS machines cost about £50. They can be used by almost anyone, although people with widespread pain may not be able to use TENS. For some people, it offers short-term pain relief when other treatments fail to do so.

Ask your doctor about TENS. If there is a pain clinic in your area, the facility may be able to lend or hire you a TENS machine. Tell your doctor if you decide to try TENS, to make sure you are a good candidate.

Biofeedback

As we learned in Chapter 1, the brain is the control centre for all pain messages. The way your cerebral cortex perceives the pain messages, sent via the peripheral nerves and the spinal cord, can depend on many things. Can the brain learn to control the way it senses pain, perhaps reducing the intensity of the pain? A treatment called *biofeedback* is based on the belief that it can.

Biofeedback is a treatment technique in which you are trained to reduce your pain by using signals from your own body. A machine picks up electrical signals in the muscles (electromyographs or EMGs). These are translated into a form you can detect: the machine triggers a flashing light bulb, perhaps, or activates a beeper every time there is an increase in your muscle activity.

When you experience pain, you may tense your muscles, which in turn may produce more pain. If you are made aware of this increased muscle activity using an EMG feedback machine, you can then use a variety of techniques to relax your muscles, all the time getting feedback via your EMG on how successful you are being. The biofeedback machine acts as a kind of sixth sense which allows you to 'see' or 'hear' activity inside your body.

This treatment is recommended for people with fibromyalgia, but is less successful in people with arthritis.

What happens during biofeedback? In biofeedback, the doctor or therapist attaches electrodes or sensors to various parts of your body, particularly areas where you might be feeling pain or tension. The electrodes are connected to a computer or other instruments that record the various reactions you have to pain: body temperature, heart rate, muscle tension or even brain waves.

Then, you'll learn some mind-control techniques, such as visualization (focusing on pleasant imagery or fantasies where you are in control of your pain), or relaxation techniques, such as deep breathing. The biofeedback equipment should be able to show you how your relaxation techniques are affecting your body's processes. The practitioner will teach you to use these techniques to control your muscles and, therefore, your heart rate and blood flow. You'll have to do this several times and practise the techniques on your own. Eventually, you should be able to do these techniques on your own and see a positive result.

Does biofeedback really work? Some research shows that it can work, and learning relaxation therapies and seeing how they can affect your pain response is a positive, risk-free treatment option. You are learning to take control of your own body and your own reaction to pain. There is evidence that biofeedback can help relieve many forms of chronic pain, such as back pain, and tension and migraine headaches.

Hydrotherapy, Water Exercise and Balneotherapy

Better known as soaking in a hot tub, Jacuzzi™ or pool spa, *hydrotherapy* seems like a natural way to massage painful muscles and joints, or to relax the body in order to reduce painful muscle tension. You can explore hydrotherapy on your own, such as in your bathtub, hot tub or home whirlpool bath; at a health spa (in fact the word 'spa' is an acronym for the Latin term *sante per aqua,* or 'health by water'); or under medical supervision at a pain clinic or rehabilitation centre.

The soothing but gentle pressure of water jets against sore, tightened or tense muscles can relieve back pain and other muscle-related pain. People with chronic pain syndromes that involve stress can find the soaking and bubbling action of the warm water relaxing. And soaking in warm or hot water is a widely recommended therapy for people with the joint pain and stiffness of arthritis. So hydrotherapy is an easy, low-risk therapy for many people in pain, something that may not completely relieve their pain but can be added as a complementary therapy to their pain-management plan. Hydrotherapy provides only temporary relief from chronic pain.

Some people cannot use hot tubs or spas, depending on their health condition. People with high blood pressure or diabetes or those taking some medicines should avoid hot tubs for health reasons. Ask your doctor if this therapy is appropriate for you and what, if any, precautions you should take. Do not mix alcohol or sedative drugs with hydrotherapy, as you could become drowsy and fall asleep in the water.

Another type of hydrotherapy is water exercise, or aquarobics, a highly recommended and widely available therapy that is easy for most people with chronic pain to do. Exercises performed in warm pools allow the person to increase flexibility, cardiovascular health and muscle strength without the pain and strain of traditional land exercise. Tell the leader about your condition so that you do not over-exercise and then feel worse when you get out of the pool.

A similar therapy that may provide warmth and relief to sore body parts is *balneotherapy*, or mud therapy. You may be familiar with mudpacks or herbal body wrap treatments at fancy spas as a way to relax the spirit. Some people also use warm mud compresses to relieve swelling and pain in joints.

Taken one step further, some people believe that the mineral-rich mud from the Dead Sea is particularly beneficial. However, the few scientific studies made of this therapy are too small to be able to draw any firm conclusions.

Whilst more research is needed to determine if the mineral content of the mud, the mud itself, or just the soothing warmth of the mud compresses helps people's painful joints feel better, this therapy may provide some temporary relief of pain or, at least, relaxation.

Hypnosis

Many people associate hypnosis with carnival entertainment or trickery. But as a serious treatment it dates back a few hundred years, and is utilized by many medical professionals. Hypnosis may be effective for some people in chronic pain. Although some people can hypnotize themselves, it may be easier at first to work with a trained professional, such as a psychiatrist, psychologist or hypnotherapist.

Hypnosis was first employed by Franz Anton Mesmer, an Austrian doctor, who used it to treat patients with various nervous conditions or ailments by lulling them into a state of extreme mental relaxation. This practice, first known as *mesmerism* after its creator, involved the person staring at a light or object until they reached this very relaxed state.

Hypnosis is done much the same way today. In this state, the person is more susceptible to suggestion, and the doctor can help the person learn to relax tense muscles or reduce the stress that may be causing or worsening pain. Hypnosis has been used as a therapy for chronic migraine headaches, as well as other painful conditions.

Ultrasound Therapy

Ultrasound or ultrasonography (see p. 41) is used extensively in diagnosis. It also may be used as a therapy: the high-frequency sound waves emit a soothing heat that may be used to relieve muscle or tissue pain. Similar to the heat therapy provided by heating pads or hydrotherapy, ultrasound offers only temporary relief.

A health-care professional (usually a physiotherapist) trained in ultrasound must administer the therapy. Doctors will usually prescribe ultrasound therapy when a person is experiencing a severe flare of pain that may not be adequately relieved by pain medicines. Ultrasound therapy is not recommended for people whose pain is accompanied by inflammation, because the heat might worsen the swelling. But for many people, ultrasound therapy is a useful complement to their pain-management treatments.

A similar type of ultrasound therapy called *shock-wave therapy* was not found to be very

beneficial in a recent Australian study, where people with the painful foot condition plantar fasciitis underwent treatment of shock or sound waves over a three-week period. In the UK, the National Institute for Health and Clinical Excellence is evaluating the value of this therapy in plantar fasciitis. Progress on the evaluation can be found on the NICE web site (see the Resources section for contact details).

Consult your doctor to see if he recommends using this therapy for your pain condition.

Prolotherapy

A relatively new experimental technique for chronic pain relief, *prolotherapy* aims to relieve pain by rebuilding and strengthening weakened connective tissues, particularly ligaments and tendons that may be painful due to injury or continued stress or pressure. Because muscles, ligaments and tendons support the bones, when they weaken you are more susceptible to pain and further injury.

Prolotherapy is often used to treat back pain, neck pain, sciatica or *whiplash*, a common and painful condition where the neck is whipped back and forth suddenly due to an impact, such as a car accident. Prolotherapy is also called sclerotherapy, proliferative injection therapy, stimulated ligament repair, regenerative injection therapy or non-surgical ligament reconstruction. As these names suggest, the therapy is meant to repair or restore the damaged or weakened connective tissues that can no longer properly support joints and bones, leading to pain with every movement. Prolotherapy is usually administered by a doctor.

Prolotherapy differs from other injection therapies, and that's why it's still controversial. In prolotherapy, the doctor injects an irritating solution into the damaged or painful soft tissues. Rather than traditional injections, which use an anti-inflammatory medication, prolotherapy's aim is to *create* inflammation. Why? Proponents of the therapy believe this intentional inflammation will increase blood circulation in the painful area and hasten the healing process. So the small tears or weaknesses in the damaged connective tissues will heal, the tissues will strengthen and the pain will subside. Normally, two or three treatments are given, with a gap of one to four weeks between them.

Prolotherapy is still controversial because there is a lack of research evidence to prove its benefit. However, a small number of randomized clinical trials have shown that it is safe, and may be effective.

Aromatherapy

Sniffing pleasant fragrances is a soothing, relaxing activity, but some people have refined this practice into a treatment called *aromatherapy*. Aromatherapy involves smelling various fragrances from essential oils (concentrated amounts of a fragrance derived from a plant), candles or incense to relax, relieve pain and reduce symptoms. Popular aromatherapy essential oils include eucalyptus, peppermint, rosemary, laurel, chamomile, marjoram, jasmine and lavender. Epsom salts or sea salts may be used in hot aromatherapy baths.

Use of aromatic herbs or incense as a way to heal physical or emotional pain dates back thousands of years. The ancient Egyptians, Chinese, Greeks, Indians and other civilizations used such practices as part of their healing rites. During the Black Death epidemic in medieval Europe, doctors felt that pestilence and disease might spread in foul-smelling air or mists, leading to a practice of wearing masks containing fragrance as a way to purify the air they breathed and protect them from disease.

In 1928, a French practitioner named Rene Maurice Gattefosse coined the term 'aromatherapy' to describe the emerging contemporary practice of using fragrance for healing. Aromatherapy has gained popularity in recent years as a method of relieving stress and healing various problems. However, the term may be misunderstood, applied too broadly or misused. Many product manufacturers use the term aromatherapy to promote any good-smelling product, from candles to room sprays to carpet deodorizers.

Aromatherapy as a pain-relief therapy involves smelling specific scents for certain purposes. You can be aided by an aromatherapy practitioner or therapist, who will administer the treatments or guide you in doing it yourself. Aromatherapy applications include massage with particular oils, steam baths with essential oils added to the steam source, aromatic baths to soak in, inhalation using a cloth or an electronic diffuser, candles, sprays, aromatic rubs or creams and more.

Aromatherapy may not provide effective relief for chronic pain, but some aromatherapy treatments may provide relaxation, easing tense muscles. Hot baths or steam baths might be soothing to sore joints and muscles, and adding the essential oil may provide some additional soothing qualities to the mind. It is important to use any of these treatments properly and with your doctor's knowledge. Some essential oils or creams that come in contact with the skin might cause rashes or other skin irritations. It's important to keep any essential oils or other fragrance sources away from the eyes, particularly sprays that might contain alcohol, chemical propellants or other irritants.

Does aromatherapy really work? Evidence does not yet support the efficacy of this therapy on its own for pain relief, but aromatherapy may provide help in achieving relaxation, leading to easing of tense muscles that can cause pain.

CONTROVERSIAL COMPLEMENTARY THERAPIES

Some other complementary treatments for chronic pain are controversial and spark a division of opinion and debate among doctors and other health-care professionals. Many of these treatments simply may not work, or they may work for some people but not for others. Some people feel that if something can't hurt, it's worth trying. That's up to you. Most therapies involve some cost as well as your time and effort. So saying 'it couldn't hurt' is really not true: if you pay for some-

thing that doesn't work and can't easily get a refund for your money, it hurts! You may also feel discouraged by the failed treatment, causing additional stress and anxiety about your chronic pain.

The best way to avoid this situation is to talk to your doctor and ask for advice. You can also conduct some of your own research on the Internet or by reading reputable health journals for reports of study results on various treatments.

Below are a few other treatments for chronic pain that could be considered to be controversial:

Low-level laser therapy. Lasers, beams of highly concentrated light, first appeared in science-fiction movies, but some doctors and physiotherapists treat painful areas of the body with low-level laser beams as a way to stimulate cell growth, boost endorphin production, treat inflammation or promote healing of damaged nerves. It remains uncertain whether this therapy really works for treating chronic pain.

Magnet therapy. The wearing or application of magnets as a method of healing or pain relief is ancient, first used by the Egyptians and Greeks. In recent years, people in pain revived the practice as a way to relieve pain, particularly after injuries, accidents, or in cases of arthritis, fibromyalgia or back pain. Magnets may be worn as a wristband or neck collar or as insoles.

The therapy aims to change the way cells

behave or to alter body chemistry to promote healing, but many doctors, scientists and sceptics claim this treatment is bogus – just a ploy to get you to buy a magnet bracelet or device. Research evidence to date cannot demonstrate any benefit from magnet therapy when compared with placebo devices. Many magnets sold in retail stores or through the Internet have no power and probably no benefit, but it is estimated that, world-wide, over £3 billion has been spent on magnet therapy. The future of magnet therapy may lie in more powerful devices that can emit a stronger form of magnetic energy, called pulse electromagnetic therapy. This therapy, rising in popularity, may be more worthwhile.

Gin-soaked raisins. Soaking raisins in gin or other alcoholic beverages and eating them is an old folk remedy for arthritis pain. The gin may offer a temporary dulling of aches, but alcohol is not recommended as a pain reliever. Although they may be tasty, gin-soaked raisins do not offer any real medical benefit.

Marijuana. Marijuana, the common name for the widely grown but illegally (in most countries) sold or used plant *Cannabis sativa,* is highly controversial as an analgesic and anti-nausea treatment. Many battles between the legal, political, medical and patient communities are taking place as some people in chronic pain fight for the option to use marijuana as a medicine. Marijuana, when smoked or ingested, can create an extreme sense of relaxation and pain relief for a time. Yet it can also be psychologically (though not physically) addictive, and is viewed negatively as a street drug. In the UK it was reclassified as a Class C drug in 2004, although it is still placed within the Misuse of Drugs Regulations as a Schedule 1 drug, implying that it has no medical use.

Some studies show that marijuana may have a positive effect on pain receptors in the brain and help to reduce the brain's pain response, similar to the way analgesic drugs work. In the UK, a cannabinoid drug called nabilone is licensed for medical use but only as an anti-sickness treatment in cancer patients receiving chemotherapy. Although nabilone is a synthetic cannabinoid, it still has many of the effects of cannabis, and may cause psychological addiction. More studies are required to determine if a medical use for marijuana in terms of chronic pain treatment merits its legalization as a substance that can be prescribed by doctors.

YOU DECIDE

Whether you wish to try a complementary treatment for your pain or just stick to more tried-and-true options, there are an increasing number of treatments available to explore. Some of these treatments are less involved or invasive than others, allowing you to try them without significant risk or cost. It's important to be fully informed before you try any complementary treatment, and to tell your doctor whatever you do. In some cases, your doctor can offer you a referral or suggestions about what treatments will work best for your type of pain, and many doctors are open to their patients creating an integrative pain-management plan.

Some treatments that lie outside the realm of drugs or surgery, but are not quite as experimental as those covered in this chapter, are what we call 'do-it-yourself' therapies or lifestyle management techniques. A person in chronic pain needs to create a healthy overall lifestyle to control their daily pain and to manage the underlying disease that causes the pain.

This concept is at the heart of any successful pain-management plan. You will probably hear your doctor tell you that pain medicines won't do the job alone – your actions are also an incredibly powerful weapon in the fight against chronic pain. Exercise, proper diet, relaxation and stress management, learning proper movement and getting proper sleep will help your body to heal injuries, restore energy, increase flexibility and lessen pain. Whilst exercising may be the last thing you want to do when you're in pain, it might be the first thing you should do each day to prevent and reduce pain.

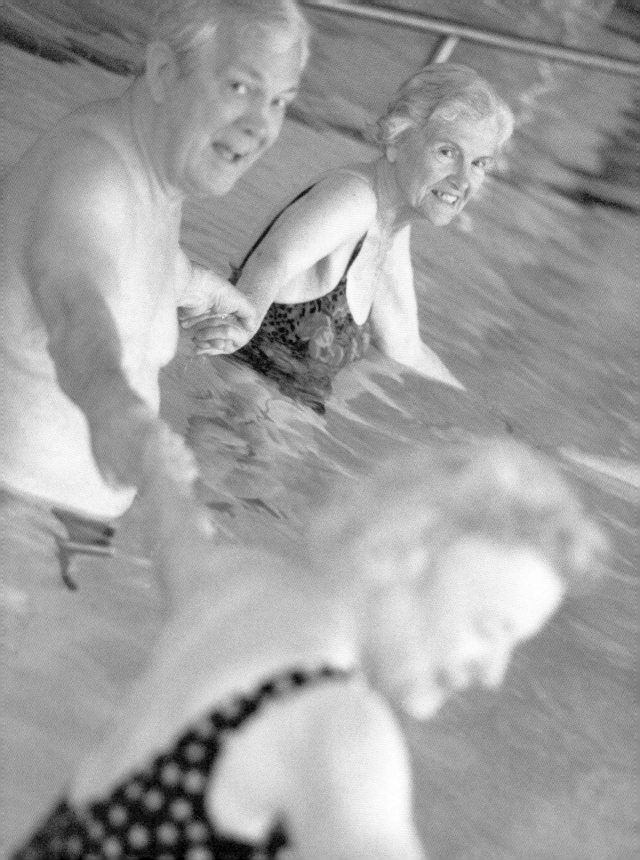

Do-It-Yourself
Pain Relief

9

CHAPTER 9: DO-IT-YOURSELF PAIN RELIEF

At the heart of every pain-management plan are not only the treatments your doctor offers – including drugs, surgery or special pain-relief therapies – but also what you can do on your own to control chronic pain and boost general health.

Many complementary treatments seek to restore the body's natural ability to heal itself. Whilst these therapies may or may not be scientifically valid, there is something basic and true in the idea behind them. When your body is working as well as it can through proper diet, exercise and stress management, it can deal better with chronic pain conditions. Muscles that are toned can better support joints weakened by arthritis. Ligaments and tendons that are flexible can promote easier, less painful movement. A mind that does not suffer from oppressive stress can promote better sleep and more relaxed muscles.

Not every pain-relief technique involves drugs or surgery, doctors or practitioners. There are many things you can do at home to provide temporary, but often noticeable, pain relief – techniques that don't cost much and can be done easily at any time. In addition, there are many methods you can try to reduce stress without having to rely on a doctor or therapist's help, although you may need professional help if your stress becomes too much for you to control on your own.

In addition to your doctor, there are health-care professionals who can help guide you in do-it-yourself pain relief and pain prevention methods. Physiotherapists can help you create a plan of exercise tailored to your physical needs and limitations. Occupational therapists can help you adjust the way you perform various activities, particularly in your home, to reduce pain and prevent injury. In addition, these professionals can prescribe braces, splints and other aids for you that may reduce pain if you are experiencing a flare-up or healing from an injury. Braces and splints can be very effective temporary help in relieving unusual episodes of pain.

First, let's discuss some easy pain-relief techniques that you can do at home. Then, we'll look at some basic principles of exercise for pain management and diet for good health. In the next chapter, we'll go over some methods you can try to reduce or control stress to keep it from worsening your pain.

THE POWER OF HEAT AND COLD

Two of the simplest, least expensive and most effective methods of pain relief are heat and cold treatments.

Heat treatments, such as heating pads or warm baths, tend to work best for soothing stiff joints and painful muscles due to arthritis, fibromyalgia or back pain. Heat helps your body get limber and ready for exercise or activity.

Cold treatments work best for flares of

pain, numbing the area and decreasing inflammation.

Try different forms of heat and cold therapy and see what works best for you.

Heat Treatments

Here are some useful tips for applying heat for pain relief.

- Take a long, very warm shower or bath first thing in the morning to ease morning stiffness, or a warm shower when you have a painful flare. Use the water jet to massage a specific, sore area, such as your lower back.
- Try thermal wraps available in many pharmacies and supermarkets. These items, which provide low-level heat over an 8-hour period, use your body heat to raise skin temperature by about 2°C.

- Try warm paraffin wax treatments, available at many health spas.
- Soak in a warm bath, hot tub or spa. Try positioning the painful area in front of the water jets for massage.
- Use a moist heating pad or make one at home by putting a wet facecloth in a freezer bag and heating it in the microwave for 1 minute. Wrap the hot pack in a towel and place it over the affected area for 15 to 20 minutes.
- Rub mineral oil on painful hands, slip on rubber washing-up gloves and place your hands in hot tap water for 5 to 10 minutes.
- Warm your clothes in the dryer before dressing each day.
- Use an electric blanket and turn it up for a few minutes before getting out of bed.

HEAT AND COLD: BE SAFE!

When using heat and cold pain therapies, avoid burns by following these guidelines:

- Use the heat or cold therapy for no more than 15 to 20 minutes at a time. Let your skin return to normal temperature before reapplying heat or cold.
- Don't place an ice or heat pack or pad directly on your skin – always use a towel or cloth in between.
- Never use analgesic creams, ointments or gels at the same time as heat treatments, as you can cause serious skin burns.
- Don't sleep with an electric heating pad on. This is a fire hazard and can also lead to excessive heating of your skin and tissues.
- Be careful using heat patches or heating pads on parts of the body that may be desensitized, such as in diabetes or other health conditions. You risk serious burns.

Cold Treatments

Here are some useful tips for applying cold for pain relief.

• Wrap a bag of ice in a towel and apply it to sore joints for about 10 minutes.

• Try cooling topical creams (containing menthol, oil of wintergreen or other cooling agents) on sore joints and muscles.

• Use a gel-filled cold pack and apply it to painful areas for about 10 minutes.

• Wrap a towel around a bag of frozen vegetables and place it on painful joints. This type of cold pack easily conforms to your joints.

• Use one of these cold treatments following exercise to soothe any sore joints or muscles.

Self-Massage

Massage given by a trained therapist can provide good pain relief, but you can also administer your own massage to sore areas of your body. Your doctor, physiotherapist or massage therapist can show you some techniques to use at home.

You can simply knead sore areas with your hands, but there are many self-massage appliances that can help you massage hard-to-reach places of the body. In addition, some people with painful hands or fingers may find it difficult to do self-massage without the assistance of a massage aid device.

Massage aids come in all styles and price ranges. At the cheaper end there are a wide variety of non-electric massage aids that have rolling rubber or wooden balls on ropes or hand-held wands. Electric hand-held massagers, which have vibrating balls or knobs that knead sore muscles, range widely in price. They come in many different styles and shapes, and may be battery-operated or plugged into an electrical outlet. Foot massage units, which can also contain warm water, also vary in price. There are car seat covers that heat up and massage your back, buttocks and thighs while driving. Full-body massage chairs can be very expensive. Whatever the price of an item, get impartial advice from a professional before buying.

Use these tips before self-massage to make the experience easier and more effective.

• Take a warm bath or shower first to relax your muscles, improve blood circulation and make your hands and fingers more supple.

• Use oil or lotion to help your hands glide over sore areas.

• Use a tennis ball or other soft rubber ball to help massage the back, buttocks, thighs or other sore areas. You can lie down, place the ball beneath the sore spot and roll against it on the floor or on a firm mattress.

Joint Protection

One of the best things you can do to prevent flares of pain or injuries that will worsen pain is to protect painful areas of your body. As you move during the course of each day, your sore, damaged joints may become stressed. We put pressure on our joints, muscles and other tissues each time we walk, lift, carry, bend down, climb stairs, twist with our hands, cut, write, reach up or do almost any other activity. You can learn ways to protect your sore joints to avoid undue pressure and further injury.

It's important to keep moving so that your body doesn't become weak and more susceptible to pain. Don't avoid activity, just use some creativity!

Here are a few things to remember:

- **Consider joint position.** Use joints in the best way to avoid excess stress. Use larger, stronger joints in your arms and legs to push or carry. For example, if you have to carry a load of groceries into the house, hug the bag with your arms and hold it close to your body so you can support the load better. Or put the bag handle over your forearm or shoulder. Don't grip the edges of the bag or the handle with your fingers. If you have to move a large object, see if you can push it with your lower body instead of trying to pull it with your hands.

- **Use helpful devices.** There are numerous appliances available to help you grab, reach, pull, push and move around. Not just canes, crutches and walkers, but also grips to add to pens and cutlery so that you can hold them with less finger stress, long-handled reachers to help you grasp items that sit high or low, and attachments to door knobs or car door handles to help you open and close doors. Use devices to help

you open containers such as tins and bottles. Select lightweight tools and appliances. Look for products designed for ease of use or make your own (such as attaching a foam-rubber hair curler to a toothbrush for easier gripping).

- **Put it on wheels.** If you have to move things from room to room, such as heavy files, laundry or gardening supplies, use a shopping bag, a rolling cart or a suitcase with wheels and a pull-up handle.

- **Ask for help if you need it.** Don't be afraid to ask family, friends or co-workers for help doing a task. Don't risk injury to your body just because you're afraid of hurting your pride.

EXERCISE: BOOST THE BODY'S DEFENCES

When you are in pain on a daily basis, the first thing you may want to do is skip your exercise routine. Who wants to work out when your body hurts? Sometimes you may feel as if you can't even get off the sofa, much less get on a treadmill or take a walk. Rest is important for people with chronic pain, but so is exercise and movement.

The second thing you may discard is your healthy diet. When you're in pain and stressed out from the pain, you may want comfort food that is easy to prepare, such as frozen pizzas or take-out Chinese noodles. But this type of diet – high in sodium, fat and calories and low in nutrients – can sap your body of energy and lessen its ability to recharge and heal.

Without the healthiest body possible (given the limitations of your chronic pain), you may be less able to handle medications or surgical procedures designed to treat your pain, leading to debilitating side effects, fatigue or lengthy recoveries after procedures. Your pain may only grow worse.

When you have chronic pain, it's important to be committed to making regular exercise and a healthy diet the cornerstone of your pain-management plan. These healthy practices, along with your medications and other treatments your doctor prescribes, can help you fight your chronic pain on a number of fronts. Pain may be caused by disease or injury, but you can more easily fight the disease, heal the injury and control the pain when you are in the best physical and emotional shape possible.

The Benefits of Exercise for Pain

If you are in pain, it can be difficult to get up and move around. You hurt, so you don't feel like moving. You feel like resting on the sofa, not riding a bike or lifting weights. So you give up exercise, and after a short period of time, your body deteriorates. You lose some flexibility or range of motion. Your muscles, unused and dormant, may weaken or *atrophy*, making them more painful and less able to support joints weakened by arthritis. Your tendons, ligaments and other connective tissues, because you are not flexing and stretching them regularly, become less flexible and more susceptible to painful tearing, strain and inflammation. Your bones, because you are not performing important weight-bearing exercises (such as walking or lifting weights), may weaken, leading to osteoporosis. People with osteoporosis are more susceptible to painful, debilitating fractures and dangerous falls.

As you can see, not exercising is a bad break in your body's cycle of good health, making chronic pain worse and lessening your ability to fight painful conditions and diseases.

All right, you know the downside of not exercising. Why will exercise help you fight chronic pain? Exercise has many proven, pain-fighting benefits. Regular exercise that contains the three basic types of movement – cardiovascular or heart-revving exercise, flexibility or range-of-motion exercises, and strengthening or muscle-and-bone-building exercise – can improve your heart and blood circulation, build stronger bones, and increase flexibility to reduce the strain on soft tissues. Exercise also boosts your brain's natural production of endorphins, those pain-fighting hormones that act much the same as analgesic medicines. Exercise can also reduce stress and anxiety, which can worsen pain or even cause painful muscle tension. Exercise can help.

Exercise can also burn calories to help you lose weight or control weight. This is an important benefit because excess pounds on your frame can add great stress to bones, joints, nerves and muscles that may be damaged or weakened due to your chronic disease. People who weigh the appropriate amount for their age, height and body style often experience less pain than those who are overweight or *obese*, extremely overweight. People who are overweight may have more problems when having surgery.

A Solid Exercise Plan

What is a good exercise programme that will help you manage your chronic pain? For one, you should exercise regularly – at least five days per week, and at least 30 minutes to an hour per day of physical activity similar in intensity to brisk walking. Don't worry if you do not exercise now – you can work up to this level slowly. In fact, most doctors or physiotherapists would not recommend that you go from doing no exercise to trying to jog three miles a day. You would only fail to complete your run, probably hurt yourself and then never want to exercise again! Start with a gentle, regular exercise routine and slowly add different components to create a comprehensive plan.

That plan should include exercises that fall into these three categories:

- **Flexibility or range-of-motion exercises:** When you stretch, bend or sway to increase mobility of joints.

- **Strengthening exercises:** When you apply force to a resistant object. Lifting weights and muscle contractions against an immovable object fall in this category.

- **Cardiovascular, aerobic or endurance exercises:** When you use large muscles at a sustained rate over a period of time, increasing your heart rate and working up a sweat. Aerobic exercise strengthens the heart, circulatory system and lungs, and includes dancing, fast walking, swimming and jogging.

All types of exercise serve to reduce stress, so if your plan starts with just one or two of the three components, you should see some stress-relief benefit. And that's good for controlling pain. As you build your exercise programme to include more techniques and longer time spent exercising, your pain-control and stress-management benefits will increase.

Can Exercise Increase Your Pain?

You may fear exercise because you think you will worsen your pain or damage your muscles and joints. This is understandable. Warming up with stretching before you exercise, and cooling down with more stretching and breathing after you exercise, will help you avoid injury or pain due to exercise.

It's important to learn the difference between the type of pain you experience from sore muscles after exercising and the type of pain caused by overuse or inflammation of joints. Sore muscles usually stem from over-stretching or overusing muscles by working out after a long period of not exercising at all. This type of pain normally begins 24–36 hours after your workout and may last for 24 to 48 hours.

If you do have exercise-related muscle pain, increase your warm-up exercises before proceeding to the rest of your exercise activity and do a full range of stretches afterwards, or scale back your programme until your muscles

ARE YOU DOING TOO MUCH?

As we said earlier in this chapter, if you don't exercise at all, start slowly as you begin working out. Increase your activity level at a gradual pace to avoid injuries or more pain – not something you want if you already have a chronic pain condition.

Look for these signs that you may be overexerting yourself:

• Increased or unusual pain that lasts for more than an hour after exercise

• Increased feelings of weakness
• Excessive fatigue after exercise
• Decreased range of motion or flexibility

If you experience any of these feelings, cut back on the amount of time you spend exercising or on the level of exertion, and talk to your doctor or physiotherapist. He or she may be able to suggest a change in your routine as well as a temporary pain-relief measure for your exercise-related pain.

become more accustomed to exercise. Once you feel that you are used to your programme, gradually increase the length and/or intensity of your workout.

When you overuse joints by exercise, usually you experience pain or swelling. If you notice these symptoms (see the box above), treat the problem by elevating the affected area, resting it and using ice packs to reduce swelling. Talk to your doctor or therapist about your exercise programme and the problems you encountered.

Some people with chronic pain may not be able to perform some exercises, but should be able to find techniques that fall into all of the above categories. Some exercises are jarring to bones and joints, or involve extreme bending or stretching that may be too painful or difficult for your condition. Don't worry! You

can achieve the same benefits from less strenuous techniques.

No matter what your situation, you should consult your doctor before beginning any exercise programme. Talk to him about your problems and needs. He should be able to suggest a beneficial and manageable exercise programme for you.

Some GPs will be able to refer you, under the Exercise Referral Scheme, to a local health club for a subsidized trial of exercise. You will be provided with a personalized exercise programme and, because most sessions are closed to the general public, you will be exercising only with people in similar circumstances. These sessions can help you find the right exercise for your ability level and pain condition.

Luckily, there are many easy and gentle exercises that you can do to begin increasing flexibility, cardiovascular health and strength – exercises that don't involve expensive club memberships, fancy equipment or a big chunk of your daily free time. In addition, there are many alternative forms of exercise that involve less sweat and strain than the traditional 'workout' but achieve many pain-management benefits. We go over some of the best pain-management exercise routines here, and also offer some gentle stretching exercises that anyone can do to increase flexibility.

Flexibility Exercises

When you have chronic pain, you might not want to move any more than necessary. Nevertheless, it is very important to stay mobile, moving all your joints through their range of motion on a regular basis. Each joint has a range of motion, which is the fullest extent you can move it in any direction. If you don't keep joints flexible through proper exercise, you could experience stiffness, immobility and more pain. Maintaining range of motion is key to having the best quality of life you can.

Flexibility or range-of-motion exercises are daily stretches designed to help you keep joints limber and mobile even if you have chronic pain. You can incorporate these stretches into your normal routine. For example, perform them in the morning after your morning shower or bath and before you get dressed for the day. Do range-of-motion stretches before any activity that may be exerting, such as a shopping trip or attending the office picnic, to keep your body limber.

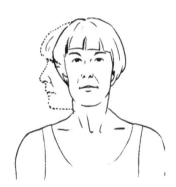

EXERCISE 1: HEAD TURNS

- LOOK STRAIGHT AHEAD.
- TURN HEAD TO LOOK OVER SHOULDER.
- HOLD THREE SECONDS.
- RETURN TO FRONT.
- REPEAT ON THE OTHER SIDE.

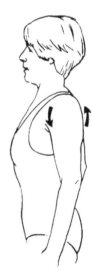

EXERCISE 2: SHOULDER CIRCLES

- MOVE SHOULDERS SLOWLY IN A CIRCULAR MOTION.

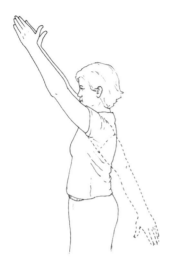

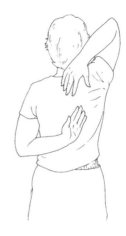

EXERCISE 3: FORWARD ARM REACH

• POSITION YOUR ARMS BEHIND YOU, PALMS FACING
  ONE ANOTHER.

• RAISE ONE OR BOTH ARMS FORWARD AND UP AS
  HIGH AS POSSIBLE (ONE ARM MAY HELP THE OTHER,
  IF NEEDED).

• LOWER ARMS SLOWLY.

EXERCISE 4: BACK PAT AND RUB

• REACH ONE ARM UP TO PAT BACK.

• REACH THE OTHER ARM BEHIND YOUR LOWER BACK.

• SLIDE HANDS TOWARD EACH OTHER.

• HOLD THREE SECONDS.

• ALTERNATE ARM POSITION.

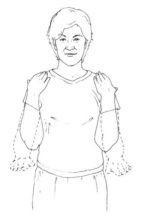

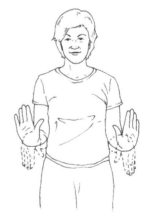

EXERCISE 5: ELBOW BEND AND TURN

• TOUCH FINGERS TO SHOULDERS, PALMS TOWARD
  YOU.

• TURN PALMS DOWN AS YOU STRAIGHTEN ELBOWS
  OUT TO SIDE.

EXERCISE 6: WRIST BEND

• STAND WITH ELBOWS TUCKED TO SIDES.

• BEND WRISTS UP.

• HOLD THREE SECONDS.

• BEND WRISTS DOWN.

• HOLD THREE SECONDS.

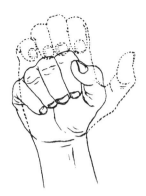

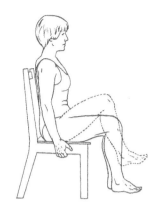

EXERCISE 7: FINGER CURL

- OPEN HAND FLAT, FINGERS STRAIGHT.
- BEND EACH JOINT SLOWLY TO MAKE A LOOSE FIST.
- HOLD THREE SECONDS.
- STRAIGHTEN FINGERS AGAIN.

EXERCISE 8: KNEE LIFT

- SIT STRAIGHT UP IN A CHAIR.
- LIFT ONE KNEE UP THREE OR FOUR INCHES OFF CHAIR.
- HOLD THREE SECONDS AND LOWER.
- REPEAT WITH OTHER KNEE (YOU MAY HELP BY LIFTING THE KNEE WITH YOUR HANDS UNDER YOUR THIGH).

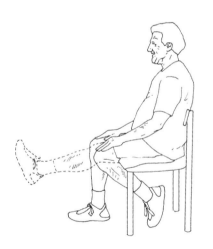

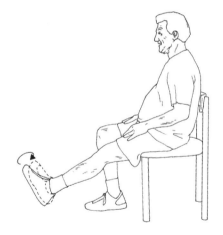

EXERCISE 9: LEG BEND AND LIFT

- SIT UP STRAIGHT IN A CHAIR.
- BEND KNEE, PUTTING YOUR HEEL UNDER THE CHAIR.
- HOLD THREE SECONDS.
- STRAIGHTEN KNEE OUT IN FRONT.
- HOLD THREE SECONDS.

EXERCISE 10: ANKLE CIRCLES

- STICK YOUR FOOT OUT AWAY FROM THE CHAIR.
- LIFT YOUR FOOT A LITTLE AND CIRCLE IT ROUND FROM THE ANKLE.
- BRING YOUR FOOT BACK TOWARDS THE CHAIR.
- REPEAT WITH THE OTHER FOOT.

Limber muscles and joints can help you maintain your balance, avoid falls and prevent injuries or aches. You can do flexibility stretches almost anywhere, including a pool and some in the bath.

Tips: Use gentle, smooth movements rather than quickly jerking your limbs, neck and other movable parts. Wear clothes that allow you to move your joints through their full range of motion with ease. Choose a place that is comfortable and gives you enough room to stretch your limbs fully.

Strengthening Exercises

There are many ways to build strength in your muscles and improve the condition of your bones, tendons and ligaments. Strengthening exercises that build muscle tone will help keep your joints stable and make movement easier. Weight training is a logical method that comes to mind as a way to build strength, but this method may not be a good choice for you if you don't exercise at all or you find weightlifting intimidating. You can build strength slowly and easily through simple

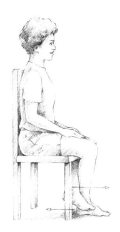

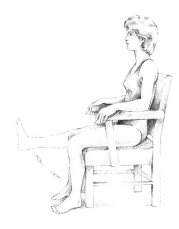

ISOMETRIC EXERCISE:

SIT IN A STRAIGHT-BACKED CHAIR AND CROSS YOUR ANKLES. YOUR LEGS CAN BE ALMOST STRAIGHT, OR YOU CAN BEND YOUR KNEES AS MUCH AS YOU LIKE. PUSH FORWARD WITH YOUR BACK LEG AND PRESS BACKWARD WITH YOUR FRONT LEG. EXERT PRESSURE EVENLY SO THAT YOUR LEGS DO NOT MOVE. HOLD AND COUNT OUT LOUD FOR SIX TO TEN SECONDS. RELAX. THEN CHANGE LEG POSITIONS AND REPEAT.

AS YOU DO THIS EXERCISE REGULARLY, YOU CAN ADD REPETITIONS (THE NUMBER OF TIMES YOU DO THE MOVE) TO BUILD MORE STRENGTH.

ISOTONIC EXERCISE:

SIT IN A CHAIR WITH BOTH FEET ON THE FLOOR AND SPREAD SLIGHTLY APART. RAISE ONE FOOT UNTIL YOUR LEG IS AS STRAIGHT AS YOU CAN MAKE IT. HOLD AND COUNT OUT LOUD FOR SIX TO TEN SECONDS. GENTLY LOWER YOUR FOOT TO THE FLOOR. RELAX. REPEAT WITH THE OTHER LEG.

AS YOU DO THIS EXERCISE REGULARLY, YOU CAN ADD REPETITIONS OR USE LIGHT ANKLE WEIGHTS (0.5– 1 KILO TO START) TO INCREASE RESISTANCE.

exercises, even moves you can do while sitting in a chair.

There are two ways in which we can strengthen our muscles: isometric exercises and isotonic exercises. In *isometric* exercises, you tense or tighten muscles, but don't move joints. In *isotonic* exercises, you concentrate on moving joints. Isotonic exercises are different from simple stretching or range-of-motion exercises (see p. 165). They emphasize building muscle strength. Opposite are sample exercises in each category.

Weight training. Whilst lifting weights may seem like an activity favoured more by young, muscle-bound men than people with chronic pain, you may be surprised to see more and more older adults lifting at your local gym. Weight training, whether with free weights (such as bar bells or dumb bells), weight machines or weighted ankle and wrist straps, is a good way to build muscle strength and tone, and increase bone density. It can also help control your weight and burn calories.

Do not lift weights without first consulting your doctor, and then work out with the supervision of a qualified exercise specialist. It's important to start with a small amount of weight and gradually build up what you lift, to prevent injury. As you build strength, you can also increase repetitions.

Cardiovascular, or Aerobic, Exercise

You know you are 'working out' when you break a sweat and feel your heart pumping a little bit. Those are two signs that you are doing aerobic, or cardiovascular, exercise, which is great for maintaining good circulation, a healthy heart and proper body weight.

Whilst most people hear the word 'aerobics' and think of people jumping around a gymnasium floor dressed in skimpy outfits, there are many gentle, easy forms of aerobic exercise. Cardiovascular exercise can include many different activities. This type of exercise should involve you moving large muscles (such as your legs) in a continuous, rhythmic movement (such as in walking) for a period of time long enough to raise your heart rate. The new government guidelines suggest 30 minutes a day of aerobic exercise on at least five days a week, although it can be divided into chunks for convenience. Doing aerobic exercises regularly will build your stamina, making it easier to do other activities with less fatigue.

Below are some fun, easy aerobic exercises you can try on your own. Be willing to experiment so your exercise routine does not become a boring routine!

Walking. Walking is arguably the cheapest, easiest, most convenient form of exercise, because you can do it almost anywhere or any time. Walking is an excellent type of cardiovascular and calorie-burning exercise for almost anyone. Walking requires no special skills except the ability to walk.

To walk regularly for exercise, you do need a safe, convenient place to walk. It may be

HELPFUL WALKING RESOURCES

Walking is probably the easiest way to exercise. You don't need any special equipment and you can do it all year round.

If you haven't been used to walking regularly, begin by walking a short distance every day or as often as possible. If there is a pool nearby, you can build up stamina and muscle strength by swimming. (Many areas have local authority swimming pools, so it isn't necessary to join a health club.)

Walking on your own can become a bit boring, so try to find a friend or neighbour who will accompany you, or join a walking club if there is one in your area.

Arthritis Care's booklet *Exercise and Arthritis* and the Arthritis Research Campaign's fold-out leaflet *Keep Moving* have helpful tips on exercising.

helpful and safer to walk with a spouse, friend or a group of neighbours. You can walk almost anytime and anywhere. Perhaps there is a walking club in your area. You should have supportive walking shoes and comfortable clothes. Shoes that are uncomfortable or not suitable for walking can actually increase your pain. See p. 171 for a walking plan.

Water Exercise. As we mentioned in the previous chapter, water exercise can be good for stiff, painful joints and sore muscles that are common in people with chronic pain conditions. Warm water supports your body while you move your joints through their range of motion, reducing your chance of muscle strain and additional pain.

Swimming and water aerobics are highly recommended as a cardiovascular workout, because little stress is placed on your joints. This is discussed in Chapter 8.

Bicycling. Riding a stationary or standard bicycle can offer aerobic exercise without placing much stress on damaged or painful hips, knees or feet. Some stationary bicycles have movable handles that exercise your upper body as well, offering additional cardiovascular benefit.

When beginning a cycling routine, don't pedal faster than 5 to 10 miles per hour. As you become fitter, increase your speed and/or add resistance. If you have knee pain or osteoarthritis of the knee, consult your doctor or physiotherapist to determine if bicycling is an acceptable exercise for you, as you may be at risk of injury. If you ride a standard bicycle, use proper safety equipment and choose a safe, well-paved route.

Dancing. Dance is a great cardiovascular exercise method that's rarely boring, because it's set to your favourite music. As old as civiliza-

Walking Progression For Fitness

The following suggested progressive walking routine should help you get your programme started and build endurance and stamina. When you can walk for a total of 10 minutes at a time (including a warm-up and cool-down period), try this progression chart to gradually build your walking fitness programme. If you can already walk for longer than 10 minutes at a time, enter the chart at your current level and progress from there.

Week	Time Duration Per Walking Session*	Frequency Per Week
1	10 minutes	3–5 times
2	15 minutes	3–5 times
3	20 minutes	3–5 times
4	25 minutes	3–5 times
5	30 minutes	3–5 times
6	30–35 minutes	3–5 times
7	30–40 minutes	3–5 times
8	30–45 minutes	3–5 times
9	30–50 minutes	3–5 times

10 and onward: Keep your walks at 30–60 minutes per session, 3–5 times per week.

Gradually increase your intensity until you are in the moderate range (if you are not doing so yet).

* Includes warm up and cool down, but not stretching.

tion itself, dance is a part of every world culture. There are many different types of dance: disco, folk, square, step, line, ballroom, ballet, tap, jazz. You can dance alone, with a partner or in a group.

To dance for fitness, all you really need is a little space, some comfortable clothes and quality shoes, and some music. There are dance classes in virtually every community, where instructors can teach you how to perform particular dance steps and monitor your progress. Dance classes can also be social, and having a set time when you dance with your friends can encourage you to keep it up. If you do wish to join a dance class, talk to the instructor beforehand about your chronic pain or health condition. You need to find a class that is suitable for your needs. Ask the instructor about what type of clothing or footwear you need in order to participate safely.

If you would rather not dance in a formal class setting, all you have to do is turn on some tunes and get moving! Your living room

Head-to-Toe Water Workout

Try these exercises at your local pool, or as part of an aquarobics class.

(1) Knee Lift
Step 1: Stand with your left side against the pool wall.
Step 2: Bend your right knee and bring your thigh parallel to the water's surface, or as high as you can. (Cup your hands behind your knee for extra support.)
Step 3: Straighten your knee, lower your leg. Repeat on the left side.

(2) Arm Circles
Step 1: Raise both arms forward a few inches below water level. (Keep elbows straight.)
Step 2: Make small circles (grapefruit size) with your arms. Increase the circles to basketball size, then decrease.
Step 3: Alternate between inward and outward circles. (Don't raise your arms out of the water or let them cross.)

(3) Side Bend
Step 1: Place your feet shoulder-width apart and relax your knees.
Step 2: Bend slowly toward the right. Return to starting position and bend to the left. (Don't bend forward or twist or turn your trunk.)
Step 3: You can try the exercise with your arms hanging at your sides, with your hand sliding down your thigh as you bend. Repeat on your left side.

(4) Ankle Bend
Step 1: Place your hands on your hips or hold the side of the pool for support.
Step 2: Bend your foot up, then down.
Step 3: Repeat with your other foot.

will do just fine for a dance floor. Or try stepping out to a local dance club with your spouse, family or friends.

Use good judgement when dancing for fitness. Don't try to push yourself to dance more vigorously, or to copy difficult steps, before you know you are ready. Wear comfortable clothing that allows you to move freely and perspire. Dancing should be a fun way to work up a sweat.

Alternative Exercise Methods

Some people find exercise boring or unpleasant. Gentle, alternative forms of exercise can seem easier and more interesting for some people. For people with chronic pain, a gentler form of exercise that still has endorphin-boosting, flexibility-increasing and aerobic benefits can seem like the best option.

It's likely that one of the following forms of exercise is taught in your area. Get instruction from a qualified professional so that you perform the exercises properly, get the most benefit from them and reduce your chances of injury or strain.

Yoga. Practised by an increasing number of people in recent years, *yoga* has been a staple exercise routine for millions of people in India for centuries. Yoga is part of the traditional Indian healing philosophy known as *Ayurveda*.

There are many types of yoga. Some forms are gentle and others are more energetic or strenuous, causing you to break into a sweat. Hatha yoga is the gentle, most common kind of yoga, and it involves gentle stretching movements and balancing exercises known as postures that condition the whole body.

Practising yoga regularly (you can do it daily) improves flexibility, balance and strength, because it involves stretching as well as bearing the weight of your body. Yoga is also relaxing and often includes meditation or deep breathing. Yoga is taught at many special centres, exercise clubs or spas, as well as through instructional tapes and videos. If you have chronic pain, learn yoga from a trained professional before trying routines on your own.

T'ai chi. In China, where *t'ai chi* began, this combination of graceful motions is considered a martial art, such as karate or tae kwon do. But t'ai chi doesn't look like fighting. Its controlled movements require grace and precision. Luckily, almost anyone can learn the simple, gentle movements of t'ai chi, gaining its health benefits.

Research studies have found that t'ai chi improves balance, reducing the risk of dangerous falls and injuries. T'ai chi is increasingly popular among people with back pain or arthritis. Explore videotapes that instruct you in the practice of t'ai chi, books about t'ai chi, or t'ai chi classes at your local adult education college and health clubs.

Qi Gong. *Qi gong* (pronounced *chee kung*) is another ancient Asian practice that aims to promote health and the body's natural healing ability. As we learned in Chapter 8, qi is the Chinese term for the natural energy flow and balance in the body.

There are several forms of qi gong, which involve meditation, breathing exercises and movements. Qi gong exercises seem less graceful than t'ai chi moves, and, like yoga, there are some more vigorous styles of qi gong. But qi gong exercises are appropriate for people of all ages and abilities, and can even be done from a bed or wheelchair.

Few studies confirm qi gong's benefits for pain relief, but one 1998 study of people with fibromyalgia who used qi gong along with meditation practices reported improvement in depression, pain and ability to function. Qi gong is taught at many local adult education centres or health clubs nationwide.

Pilates. The *Pilates* method of exercise started in the 1920s, and it's becoming increasingly popular. Pilates conditions and strengthens the body through specific exercises that emphasize proper body alignment, injury prevention and breathing.

Whilst other exercises may focus on various parts of the body or on the body as a whole, Pilates really concentrates on the role of the back and spine in overall health. Pilates exercises may be difficult to perform at first, which is why it's essential to receive proper instruction and supervision in this technique. Pilates involves strengthening and stretching exercises to develop the muscles in the lower back and abdomen so they can provide firm support for your whole body's movements. Pilates aims to promote proper spinal alignment and stability. Usually taught in special Pilates centres or classes at health clubs, you often perform the exercises on a special bench-like piece of equipment.

As we have learned, managing your chronic pain isn't simple – it requires a comprehensive approach from you and your doctor. Managing your pain can require making positive changes to your lifestyle, including improving your diet, quitting bad habits such as smoking, taking your medications as prescribed and getting proper rest and exercise.

One factor that may increase your pain, even if you do all of those healthful things, is stress. In the next chapter, we look at how stress may play a role in chronic pain, and offer strategies for keeping stress at bay.

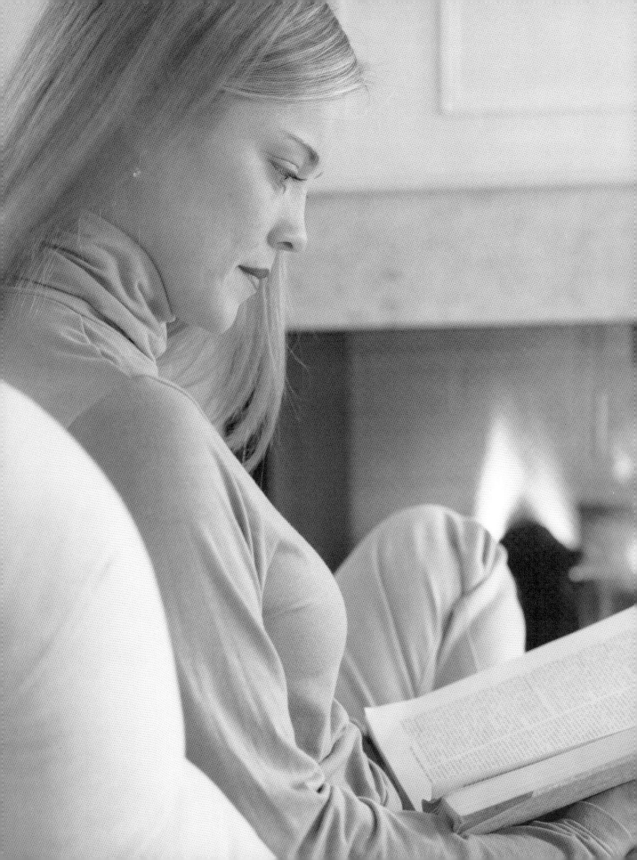

Reducing Painful Stress

10

CHAPTER 10: REDUCING PAINFUL STRESS

I't's a proven fact: Stress can make pain worse. Stress may also cause pain in some cases.

How does this happen? When you are 'stressed out', your muscles tense, causing pain. Your heart rate increases. In reaction to stress, your body secretes the hormone *adrenaline*. Adrenaline, which comes from the adrenal glands above the kidneys, is your body's natural response mechanism to a frightening or dangerous situation. But when you have constant or regular stress, your body continues to pump adrenaline. It never shuts off, and your body cannot recover from a heightened emergency state. This stressed-out state is exhausting.

For someone with chronic pain due to arthritis, fibromyalgia, back pain, nerve damage or other diseases, this constant state of stress can be dangerous. This state of emergency puts a strain on your heart, lungs and other organs. When you are in constant stress, adding to your chronic pain, you may seek out alcohol, cigarettes or drugs, abusing these substances in an unhealthy, dangerous way.

So controlling stress is vital for someone in chronic pain. Learning to relax – something that seems simple but actually requires concentration and effort – could change your life.

WHAT IS STRESS?

'Stress' has become one of the most common buzzwords of our time. Almost everyone mentions stress on a daily basis: 'I'm so stressed out at work from the pressure to make higher sales.' 'I'm having so much stress because my mother-in-law is coming to town for a visit.' 'The bills keep piling up and it's causing me to feel stressed.' Stress is something you feel all over, both in your mind and in your body.

A person with chronic pain is highly susceptible to stress and its effects. Chronic pain never lets up, so the person in pain may feel overwhelmed by their condition and feel hopeless. Family members and friends may grow impatient or intolerant of the person's condition and not offer the support necessary, adding to the stress. It may be more difficult for a person with chronic pain to keep up with their job requirements or goals, leading to even more stress.

Stress is defined as mental or physical tension, and it affects a person both mentally and physically in many cases. Stress causes mental reactions such as anxiety, worry, fear, anger and nervousness. When stressed, you might snap at someone without meaning to act that way. Stress can also cause strong physical reactions, such as stomach upset, headaches, muscle tension or pain, perspiration, heart palpitations, tightened jaw and teeth grinding. Stress can lead you to engage in unhealthy practices, such as overeating, smoking, drinking alcohol or abusing drugs. So stress is a serious health threat, and needs to be addressed as such.

Stress may be caused by mental anxiety, tension or pressure, but the reactions can be physical in nature. When we face stress from any source, our bodies respond by releasing hormones such as adrenaline and cortisol into the bloodstream. These hormones increase your heart rate and blood pressure and tense muscles. Why? This physical reaction probably stems from the earliest stages of human evolution, when humans faced life-or-death dangers on a regular basis. To respond to dangerous situations, they developed a physical emergency response system: the hormones released would put their whole bodies on alert status, something now called the 'fight or flight response'. In this state, we are intensely aware of the danger and ready to fight with all our might or run like crazy to survive.

This kind of response works most of the time. The stress response is beneficial during real emergencies or high-pressure situations. When the stressful situation is over, the body's vital signs should return to normal levels. Sometimes, as in the case with many people in chronic pain, they do not.

Stress levels in our modern society often remain high for sustained periods of time. You may experience stress daily from your job, traffic, your family or your health problems. If you can't release the tension after a stressful situation (such as being stuck in traffic), your body may begin to respond to every slightly stressful situation as if it's an emergency. This constant stress can wear you down both physically and mentally. Just as it's bad for your car to 'race the engine' constantly, it's bad for your body to race without a break.

People in chronic pain don't get a break from their pain and other symptoms. They may not sleep well, so they can't recharge their energy stores. Day after day, it becomes more difficult to deal with life in a positive, healthy way. You may find yourself reaching the resulting 'overload'. You could become more accident-prone. You might make more mistakes than usual. You might find it impossible to get a good night's sleep. These are signs that you need to try to relieve some of the stress in your life. Without releasing the tension and getting good sleep, your pain will feel worse.

EASING STRESS STEP BY STEP

Relaxation needs to occur one step at a time. You have to learn methods of relaxation that work for you. Understandably, you may encounter problems that make it impossible to avoid stress. Nobody can avoid stress completely. When you have health problems, you can find even ordinary challenges very stressful. You may find it difficult to calm down after you have resolved the challenge. You might find yourself getting angry with family members, friends, co-workers, your doctor or even your pain itself.

But learning and practising techniques for relaxation can help you manage stressful episodes in a healthier way. This chapter contains some proven techniques for healthy relaxation. You will have to practise them on your own, and find what works for you. Your doctor may be able to suggest methods to help you fight stress. Some complementary treatments can help reduce stress too.

The first step in controlling stress is to recognize the causes of stress. This is called *identifying stressors*. Stressors are the actual triggers to your stress. They can be anything, even supposedly joyful or simple things: visits from relatives for the holidays, leading a meeting at work, going to the doctor, meeting your daughter's new fiancé for the first time, packing for a trip, taking your car for a repair. Often, the stressor is not something you pinpoint right away. You may tell yourself that you don't mind certain tasks or activities, when in fact you do find the situation or activity stressful. For example, you may love going on a vacation with your family. But when you think about it – getting to the airport, going through check-in and security, waiting for your flight to be called, getting on the plane – these are all stressful. So these aspects of travel cause you to become tense.

The second step is recognizing how you respond to stress. These are the *reactions to the stressor*. Because stressors may not always be obvious to you, linking your physical or emotional reactions may be difficult also. For example, you may have headaches on occasion. Are these headaches caused by a stressor? Write down when you have headaches so that you can note patterns. Do you get one every time you face a stressful situation? If so, stress may be causing the headaches, not your drugs or your allergies. Keeping a journal may help you identify what causes your stress and how you respond to it.

After you identify what causes your stress and how you respond to stress, the third step is to develop coping strategies, so you deal with stress more effectively and avoid or reduce your reactions. There are many unhealthy strategies for coping with stress: smoking, drinking, abusing drugs, shouting, fighting, self-blame, avoidance. These strategies may be easy ways to 'deal' with stress in your life, but they will only increase your tension, damage your relationships and, eventually, worsen your pain.

Find coping strategies that are positive, healthy and effective. This chapter contains some suggested coping strategies to help you. You may have to experiment to find the one that works for you.

Stress Journal

You might be able to eliminate stress by learning what causes it and how you respond to it, both physically and emotionally. Physical reactions might include headaches, stomachaches, muscle tension or breaking out into a sweat. Emotional reactions might include anxiety, panicking, getting angry or crying.

By keeping a daily stress journal for a week or two, you'll discover patterns in your stress and the reactions or symptoms of stress. Once you know what causes your stress and how you react to it, you will know when you need to apply the stress-reduction methods discussed in this chapter.

Try keeping your own stress journal (see sample opposite). Write down not only what situations cause your stress, but how you felt before, during and after the situation. Does your chronic pain make you feel worried

Sample Stress Journal

Date	Time	Cause of Stress	Physical Symptoms	Emotional Symptoms
18/4	7 a.m.	Cooking breakfast for children	Fast heartbeat, tightening back muscles	Feel rushed
18/4	8 a.m.	Stuck in traffic	Headache, heart beating	Screamed at other cars
23/4	1 p.m.	Presentation for boss	Fast heartbeat, dry throat, back pain afterward	Anxious, nervous

about your job performance? Do you feel that your family and friends don't understand your pain, so you become anxious before social outings? Do you become uncontrollably angry in traffic, honking your horn continuously? Does your heart beat faster? All of these facts, when you write them in your journal, will begin to show patterns in your feelings and behaviours. You may wish to share this journal with your doctor or therapist and discuss what responses you can try.

Learning To Relax

Relaxation therapies can be done almost anywhere and at any time. Some may be more appropriate for times when you are at home and have more time to truly relax. Relaxation is not just kicking off your shoes with a beer and the TV remote control. Relaxation is a more organized, strategic activity designed to bring your body processes such as heartbeat back to normal. You will learn to relax your muscles and reduce excess pain.

Here we share a few successful stress-management techniques. Try them and see what works for you.

Deep Breathing. To practise deep breathing, sit in a comfortable chair with your feet on the floor and your arms at your sides. Close your eyes and breathe in deeply, saying to yourself , 'I am . . .,' then slowly breathe out, while saying, '. . . relaxed'.

Continue to breathe slowly, silently repeating something to yourself such as, 'My hands . . . are warm; my feet . . . are warm; my breathing . . . is deep and smooth; my heartbeat . . . is calm and steady; I feel calm . . . and at peace.'

Always coordinate the words you speak with your breathing.

Distraction techniques. Distraction techniques aim to teach your mind to focus on something other than your stress. Your mind kicks into a subconscious response pattern when you experience a stressful episode. This pattern includes physical and emotional reactions to stress and pain. But you can learn to control your mind so this response mechanism is interrupted. This does not mean that you will ignore the stress, only that you can learn to put it in perspective and therefore cope better with it.

By reading your stress journal, identify common causes of your stress: morning commuting traffic, doctor's appointments, parent/teacher conferences, phone conversations with your mother-in-law. You know these things cause stress and you know how you typically react. So anticipate the stress and think how you will handle it. Create a strategy for what you will do once the stressful situation is over – such as going window-shopping, taking a hot bath or going for a walk with your dog. Or try imagining something really pleasant during the stressful episode. Perhaps you can think about happy times spent with your family, or dream holidays you would love to take, or your favourite football team winning the Cup. You may feel, at the time, as if the problem will last forever. It won't! By thinking of the enjoyable and relaxing things you will do afterwards, you can distract your mind from the stress.

Guided Imagery. Guided imagery techniques also distract you from your stress. You can do them anywhere – on the bus, at home or in your doctor's waiting room. Or you can play special tapes that guide you

To practise guided imagery, close your eyes, take a deep breath and hold it for several seconds. Breathe out gradually, feeling your body relax as you breathe.

Think about a place you have been where you felt safe, pain-free and comfortable. Imagine it in as much detail as possible: the sounds – waves crashing against the sand, seagulls calling overhead, the wind blowing. Think of smells, tastes and sights – saltwater breezes, soft sand between your toes, coconut-scented lotion, the warm sun on your face.

Try to recapture and retain the positive feelings you had in this pleasant place and time. Remember them and keep them in your mind. Use this image to help you through painful or stressful times. Take several deep breaths and enjoy feeling calm and peaceful for a few minutes. Open your eyes.

Progressive Relaxation. This is a therapy in which the body's muscles, from head to toe, are progressively tensed and then relaxed. Progressive relaxation is a popular form of stress management, and it can also help you relax tight, tense muscles that make pain worse. Progressive relaxation is very useful for people in chronic pain. You may wish to do some basic flexibility or stretching exercises first so your muscles and tissues are properly limber.

Close your eyes and take a deep breath, filling your chest and breathing all the way down to your abdomen.

Breathe out, letting your stress flow out with the air.

Start with your feet and calves. Slowly tense your muscles. Hold for several seconds, then release the flex and relax your muscles. Gradually work your way through your major muscle groups using the same technique: upper legs, buttocks, stomach and torso, upper arms, lower arms and fingers, shoulders and neck, then to your jaw and face.

Continue breathing deeply and enjoy the feeling of relaxation before opening your eyes.

Visualization. Visualization is a technique that is very similar to distraction and guided imagery. When you have chronic pain, you often feel out of control. Pain and disease seem to control your life. Visualization techniques help reduce your stress and pain by allowing you to imagine yourself in control. You visualize yourself as the one in charge, and imagine yourself doing the things you love to do but often feel you cannot do. For example, visualize climbing a mountain or winning a marathon. By focusing on doing the things you want to do and enjoy doing, you are not focusing on the things that cause you stress.

Visualization exercise 1: Concentrate on something pleasant from your past, like the beach scene discussed before. Or imagine a new and better situation. It's creative fantasizing: Imagine yourself as a movie star accepting an award or making the big, lucrative deal at work.

Visualization exercise 2: Concentrate on symbols that represent your pain or stress in different parts of your body. Imagine that painful back muscles are bright red. Then, visualize them as turning gradually into cool, soothing blue.

Visualization exercise 3: Concentrate on an image of your pain as a little green monster. Lock the monster in a metal rubbish bin. Shut the lid, lock it and put it in a skip to be hauled away.

Sample Relaxation Exercises

Here are some useful relaxation exercises to help you control stress and pain. First, find a comfortable, safe, quiet place to perform the exercise. Focus on your breathing. Concentrate on fresh breaths coming in and tension breathing out.

Then try one or more of these exercises. If you find one that really works for you, do it any time you feel stressed or in pain.

Pain Drain. Feel within your body and note where you experience pain or tension. Imagine that the pain or tension is turning into a liquid substance. This heavy liquid flows down through your body and out through your fingers and toes. Allow the pain to drain from your body in a steady flow. Now imagine that a gentle stream flows down over your head . . . and further dissolves the pain . . . into a liquid that continues to drain away. Enjoy the sense of comfort and well-being that follows.

Disappearing Pain. Notice any tension or pain that you are experiencing. Imagine that the pain takes the form of an object, or of several objects. It can be fruit, pebbles, crystals or anything else that comes to mind. Pick up each piece of pain, one at a time, and place it in a magic box.

As you drop each piece into the box, it dissolves into nothingness. Now, again survey your body to see if any pieces remain, and remove them. Imagine that your body is lighter now, and allow yourself to experience a feeling of comfort and well-being. Enjoy this feeling of tranquillity and repose.

Healing Potion. Imagine you are in a pharmacist's that is stocked with bottles and jars of exotic potions. Each potion has a special magical quality. Some are of pure white light, others are lotions, balms and creams, and yet others contain healing vibrations. As you survey the many potions, choose one that appeals to you. It may even have your name on the container.

Open the container and cover your body with that magical potion. As you apply it, let any pain or tension slowly melt away, leaving you with a feeling of comfort and well-being. Imagine that you place the container in a special spot and that it continually renews its contents for future use.

Writing Your Stress Away

Many people use a diary to record their feelings or thoughts about their life. The practice of writing down your fears, hopes, dreams and beliefs can be fun, but it can also help you control stress. How? When you write out your feelings, you can put things in perspective, identify problems and solutions, and see patterns in your behaviour and in your life that you can change for the better.

Research supports the idea that writing in a diary can help you cope with the stress and pain of chronic illness. One study of people with rheumatoid arthritis showed that those who regularly wrote about their most stressful life events experienced a 28 per cent reduction in overall disease symptoms.

Stress can contribute to disease activity. This study also shows that reducing stress – specifically by writing about emotionally troubling events or issues – may decrease the severity of your disease. Here are some tips for starting your own diary.

- **Choose pen and paper – or a screen.** Find a bound diary with a pretty cover, a handy spiral notebook, or a blank tablet with lots of open space to write in. Or, if you prefer a computer, start a private file of documents and add pictures or choose particular fonts and colours that suit you.

- **Don't worry about grammar or spelling.** Your diary is for your eyes only. Make sure family members know that this journal is not to be read by them. You don't need to impress anyone with handwriting, proper grammar or spelling. Use a thesaurus or dictionary if you find it helpful, but don't worry about expressing your thoughts in any way other than how you normally do.

- **Choose a relaxing time and place to write regularly.** Don't try to write in your diary while you're cooking dinner for the family. Pick a time and place with few distractions so you can write without being interrupted. This time is for you alone.

- **Let it flow.** Express your emotions freely. No one else will have to see what you write, so don't be afraid to express your emotions no matter what they are.

- **Get help if you need it.** Writing in your diary may stir painful feelings. If you find these emotions difficult to deal with, consider turning to someone who can help. Your pain and stress may be too much for you to handle alone. Your doctor may refer you to a psychologist or therapist, or you can consult a counsellor, minister, rabbi or other trained clergyman. Take your diary to counselling sessions if you like, and share certain feelings you would like to discuss.

Stress doesn't have to take over your life. It's hard enough to handle daily life and responsibilities with chronic pain. You have a lot to juggle – medications, doctor's visits, family and friends, job, bills and pain. Constant stress will only make things worse, and could even seriously hurt you physically and emotionally. Avoid tense situations or aggravating people if you can. Try the techniques outlined in this chapter to learn to relax, or get help if you need it. Stress can be managed just as pain can be managed: with your effort and with help from those around you.

CONCLUSION

Chronic pain is a serious and growing problem in our society. Despite advances in medicine and understanding of the human body, many people are in poor general health and experiencing pain. Thankfully, there is hope.

There are new, powerful medications designed to attack the causes of disease and pain. There are useful, natural strategies to help people reduce their own pain and relax during stressful times. There is new research on how to eat healthily, lose weight and exercise to achieve the maximum state of fitness no matter how old you are. There are organizations that offer helpful resources for people in chronic pain, resources that include health information, exercise courses, lifestyle management classes, support groups, social outings and 24-hour web sites where you can talk to others in chronic pain and experts with answers to medical questions. The Internet has made a wealth of pain-management and health information available to almost everyone, everywhere, at any time.

Reach out in your own community and find helpful resources and guidance for living with pain. Ask your doctor for advice or strategies to help manage your pain. Learn more about the cause of your pain and what new medical advances may help you treat your pain more effectively. If you find new research and want to know more, ask your doctor. Keep up to date with studies about complementary treatments or new drugs to see what works and what may be a waste of time.

Educating yourself, dedicating yourself to good health habits and maintaining an open dialogue with your health-care professionals are three key steps to managing your pain. Whilst it would be great if a magic pill could erase your pain, in most cases that won't happen. But there are many things you can do to manage your pain and live a fuller, more active life. Pain doesn't have to win this battle – with the strategies in this book and others on the horizon, it's our hope that you will win and have a happy, less painful life.

Resources

Arthritis Care

Arthritis Care is the largest UK-wide voluntary organisation working with and for all people with arthritis. We aim to promote independence and empower people with arthritis to live positive lives as well as raise awareness of the condition. We have over 300 branches and groups, and over 70,000 supporters.

Arthritis Care:

- provides a helpline service by email, telephone and letter, weekdays 10am–4pm on a freephone helpline (0808 800 4050). Email: Helplines@arthritiscare.org.uk

- offers The Source, a helpline service for young people with arthritis and their families by telephone, letter and email. Freephone: 0808 808 2000 weekdays 10am–4pm Email: thesource@arthritiscare.org.uk

- produces a range of helpful publications including:
  a bi-monthly magazine, *Arthritis News*
  Understanding Arthritis
  Living with Osteoarthritis
  Living with Rheumatoid Arthritis
  Drugs and Complementary Therapies
  Coping with Pain
  Surgery
  Exercise and Arthritis
  Food for Thought
  Working with Arthritis
  Coping with Emotions
  Our Relationships, Our Sexuality
  Reaching Independence
  To order, call 020 7380 6540; or download from our web site: **www.arthritiscare.org.uk**

- offers a range of self-management and personal development training courses for people with arthritis of all ages to enable people to be in control of their arthritis

- runs four hotels in the UK

- campaigns for greater awareness of the needs of all people with arthritis

- has a network of staff and volunteers across the UK, and has offices in England, Wales, Scotland and Northern Ireland. Phone 020 7380 6540 to find your nearest one.

Useful Addresses

Action on Pain
20 Necton Road
Little Dunham PE32 2DN
Helpline: 0845 603 1593 (Mon–Fri, 9am–5pm)
Tel: 01760 725993
Web site: www.action-on-pain.co.uk
Provides support for people with chronic pain, and their families or carers.

Arthritis Care
18 Stephenson Way
London NW1 2HD
Helplines: 0800 800 4050
(Mon–Fri, 10am–4pm)
Helpline for young people and their families:
0808 808 2000 (Mon–Fri, 10am–2pm)
Fax: 020 7380 6505
Web site: www.arthritiscare.org.uk
Provides information and support to enable people to live with and manage arthritis. Campaigns for greater awareness and better services. The helpline is the first port of call for anyone with arthritis.Many small organisations for particular types of arthritis; for details ring the helpline on Freephone 0808 800 4050.

Arthritis Care Northern Ireland
115 Enkalon Business Park
25 Randalstown Road
Antrim BT41 4LJ
Tel: 028 9448 1380
Website: www.arthritiscare.org.uk/northernireland
The Northern Ireland branch of Arthritis Care.

Arthritis Foundation of Ireland
1 Clanwilliam Square
Grand Canal Quay
Dublin 2
Ireland
Tel: 00 353 1 66 18188
Fax: 00 353 1 66 18261
Web site: www.arthritis-foundation.com
General information and support with educational lectures. Local support groups run information and fundraising events.

Arthritis Research Campaign
Copeman House
St Mary's Court
St Mary's Gate
Chesterfield S41 7TD
Tel: 01246 558 033
Fax: 01246 558 007
Web site: www.arc.org.uk
Finances an extensive programme of research and education in a wide range of arthritis and rheumatism problems, including back pain. Has useful booklets explaining related problems and ways of coping with them.

BackCare
16 Elmtree Road
Teddington TW11 8ST
Tel: 020 8977 5474
Fax: 020 8943 5318
Web site: www.backcare.org.uk
Information and advice for people with back pain. Funds patient-orientated scientific research into the causes, treatment and prevention of back pain. Has local support groups throughout the country with regular meetings.

British Acupuncture Council
63 Jeddo Road
London W12 9HQ
Tel: 020 8735 0400
Fax: 020 8735 0404
Web site: www.acupuncture.org.uk
*Professional body offering lists of qualified
acupuncture therapists.*

British Chiropractic Association
Blagrave House
17 Blagrave Street
Reading
Berks RG1 1QB
Tel: 0118 950 5950
Fax: 0118 958 8946
To find a member chiropractor near you.

British Complementary Medicine Association
PO Box 5122
Bournemouth BH8 0WG
Tel: 0845 345 5977
Website: www.bcma.co.uk
*Maintains a register of suitably qualified
practitioners of complementary medicine.*

British Homeopathic Association
Hahnemann House
29 Park Street West
Luton LU1 3BE
Tel: 08704 443 950
Fax: 08704 443 960
Web site: www.trusthomeopathy.org
*Professional body offering lists of qualified
homoeopathic practitioners.*

British Pain Society
21 Portland Place
London W1B 1PY
Tel: 020 7631 8870
Website: www.britishpainsociety.org
*Has general information on chronic pain, and
details of pain clinics in the UK. Publishes the
booklet* Understanding and Managing Pain.

British Sjögren's Syndrome Association
PO Box 10867
Birmingham B16 0ZW
Helpline: 0121 455 6549 (Mon–Thu,
9.30am–4.30pm)
Tel (admin): 0121 455 6532 (Mon–Fri,
9am–5pm)
Web site: www.bssa.uk.net
*Self-help group giving information and advice on
how to alleviate the symptoms of Sjögren's syndrome;
publishes a quarterly newsletter.*

Carers UK
20–25 Glasshouse Yard
London EC1A 4JS
Helpline: 0808 808 7777 (Mon–Fri, 10am–noon;
2–4pm)
Tel: 020 7490 8818
Fax: 020 7490 8824
Web site: www.carersonline.org.uk
*Provides a wide range of information and support to
all carers.*

Chartered Society of Physiotherapy
14 Bedford Road
London WC1R 4ED
Tel: 020 7306 6666
Fax: 020 7306 6611
Web site: www.csp.org.uk
*For information about all aspects of physiotherapy;
offers list of chartered physiotherapists in your area.*

Children's Chronic Arthritis Association
Ground Floor
Amber Gate
City Wall Road
Worcester WR1 2AH
Tel: 01905 745 595
Fax: 01905 745 703
Web site: www.ccaa.org.uk
Offers practical information to maximise choices and opportunities and raise awareness of childhood arthritis in the community. A support network run by parents offers emotional support; runs a yearly family week-end conference.

**CHOICES for Families
of Children with Arthritis**
PO Box 58
Hove
East Sussex BN3 5WN
Web site: www.kidswitharthritis.org
Provides information for children with arthritis and their families about living with arthritis. Also provides an education resource to enhance health and social care, community and education services.

Coventry Pain Clinic
Website: www.coventrypainclinic.org.uk
Information for pain sufferers and their carers, to help people improve their pain management and coping abilities.

Department of Health
PO Box 777
London SE1 6HX
Helpline: 0800 555 777
Tel: 020 7210 4850
Textphone: 020 7210 3000
Fax: 01623 724 524
Web site: www.doh.gov.uk
Produces literature about all health issues, including prescription charges and prepayment certificates, available via the Helpline. A more technical site, with National Service Frameworks, is available at www.doh.gov.uk/nsf/arthritis

Department for Work and Pensions
Benefits Enquiry Line: 0800 88 22 00
Tel: 020 7712 2171
Textphone: 0800 24 33 55
Fax: 020 7712 2386
Web site: www.dwp.gov.uk
Government department giving information about, and claim forms for, all state benefits.

Disability Alliance
Universal House
88–94 Wentworth Street
London E1 7SA
Helpline: 020 7247 8765 (Mon & Wed, 2–4pm)
Tel: 020 7247 8776 (voice and textphone)
Fax: 020 7247 8763
Web site: www.disabilityalliance.org
Information on welfare benefits entitlement, to people with disabilities, their families, carers and professional advisers. Services include advice, campaign work, research and training.

Disabled Living Centres Council
Redbank House
4 St Chad's Street
Manchester M8 8QA
Tel: 0161 834 1044
Textphone: 0161 839 0885
Fax: 0161 839 0802
Web site: www.dlcc.org.uk
For a Centre near you, where you can see furniture, aids and equipment for elderly and disabled people. Offers training courses for health professionals; information leaflets available on request.

Disabled Living Foundation
380–384 Harrow Road
London W9 2HU
Helpline: 0845 130 9177
Tel: 020 7289 6111
Textphone: 020 7432 8009
Fax: 020 7266 2922
Web site: www.dlf.org.uk
Provides information to disabled and elderly people on all kinds of equipment in order to promote their independence and quality of life.

European League against Rheumatism (EULAR)
Eular Executive Secretariat
Witikonerstrasse 15
CH 8032 Zurich, Switzerland
Tel: + 41 1 383 9690
Fax: + 41 1 383 9810
Web site: www.eular.org
Publishes journals, holds international conferences; web site shows images of different diseases. Provides up-to-date information for professionals and patient organizations.

Expert Patients Programme
Tel: 0845 606 6040
Website: www.expertpatients.nhs.uk
To find out about becoming an 'expert patient'.

Fibromyalgia Association UK
PO Box 206
Stourbridge DY9 8YL
Tel: 0870 220 1232
Fax: 0870 752 5118
Web site: www.fibromyalgia-associationuk.org
Provides information for patients with fibromyalgia and has a network of local support groups throughout the UK. Campaigns for a better recognition and awareness of the disorder.

General Chiropractic Council
44 Wicklow Street
London WC1X 9HL
Tel: 020 7713 5155
Fax: 020 7713 5844
Website: www.gcc-uk.org
The regulatory body for chiropractors.

General Osteopathic Council
Osteopathy House
176 Tower Bridge Road
London SE1 3LU
Tel: 020 7357 6655
Fax: 020 7357 0011
Web site: www.osteopathy.org.uk
Regulatory body that offers information to the public and lists of accredited osteopaths.

Independent Living Fund
PO Box 7525
Nottingham NG2 4ZT
Helpline: 0845 601 8815
Tel: 0115 942 8191
Fax: 0115 945 0948
Web site: www.ilf.org.uk
May provide top-up funding for very severely disabled people to buy in extra personal and/or domestic care. Applicants must already be receiving the higher care allowance and at least £200 care package from Social Services. Referral via Social Services.

Institute for Complementary Medicine
PO Box 194
Tavern Quay
London SE16 7QZ
Tel: 020 7237 5156
Website: i-c-m.org.uk
For a list of qualified practitioners, send a large s.a.e. stating the therapy.

JOINTZ
Janet Harper (Sec.)
7 Newtown Heights
Newtownards BT23 7YG
Tel: 028 7982 0369
Arthritis Care's Parent Group in Northern Ireland.

Joint Zone
Web site: www.jointzone.org.uk
Free educational web site, funded by the Arthritis Research Campaign, International League of Associations for Rheumatology and others, intended mainly for medical students, with information about various forms of arthritis and treatments. Gives case studies and lectures.

Lupus UK
St James House
Eastern Road
Romford
Essex RM1 3NH
Tel: 01708 731251
Fax: 01708 731252
Web site: www.lupusuk.com
Offers support, advice and information for people with systemic lupus erythematosus.

MAVIS (Mobility Advice and Vehicle Information Service)
Department for Transport
Crowthorne Business Estate
Old Wokingham Road
Crowthorne
Berkshire RG45 6XD
Tel: 01344 661000
Fax: 01344 661066
Web site: www.mobility-unit.dft.gov.uk
Government department offering driving and vehicle assessments and advice for people with mobility problems. Can advise on vehicle adaptations for both drivers and passengers.

Motability
Goodman House
Station Approach
Harlow
Essex CM20 2ET
Helpline: 01279 635 666 (Mon–Fri, 8.45am–5.15pm)
Tel: 01279 635 999 (admin)
Textphone: 01279 632 273
Fax: 01279 632 000
Web site: www.motability.co.uk
Advises people with disabilities about powered wheelchairs, scooters, and new and used cars, how to adapt them to their needs and how to obtain funding via the Mobility Scheme.

National Ankylosing Spondylitis Society (NASS)
PO Box 179
Mayfield
East Sussex TN20 6ZL
Tel: 01435 873 527
Fax: 01435 873 027
Web site: www.nass.co.uk
Provides information and advice to patients with ankylosing spondylitis, their families and professionals. Has over 100 branches providing supervised physiotherapy one evening a week. Video and cassette tapes of physiotherapy exercises available.

National Centre for Independent Living
250 Kennington Lane
London SE11 5RD
Tel: 020 7587 1663
Textphone: 020 7587 1177
Fax: 020 7582 2469
Web site: www.ncil.org.uk
Provides advice on independent living and Direct Payments, and details of your local Centre for Independent Living, to enable people to buy private personal and/or domestic care instead of receiving it via the local authority.

NHS Direct
Tel: 0845 46 47
Textphone: 0845 606 4647
NHS24 (Scotland): 0800 22 44 88
Web site: www.nhsdirect.nhs.uk
First point of contact to find out about NHS services and for any health advice, which is available 24 hours daily, 365 days a year.

National Institute for Health and Clinical Excellence (NICE)
Website: www.nice.org.uk
The independent organization responsible for providing national guidance on the promotion of good health and the prevention and treatment of ill-health.

National Osteoporosis Society
Camerton
Bath
Somerset BA2 0PJ
Helpline: 0845 450 0230
Tel: 01761 471 771
Fax: 01761 471 104
Web site: www.nos.org.uk
Provides information and advice on all aspects of osteoporosis, the menopause and hormone replacement therapy. Encourages people to take action to protect their bones. Helpline staffed by specially trained nurses. Has local support groups.

Pain Society
21 Portland Place
London W1B 1PY
Tel: 020 7631 8870
Fax: 020 7323 2015
Web site: www.painsociety.org
Primarily for health care professionals; publishes Understanding and Managing Pain *for patients.*

Patients Association
PO Box 935
Harrow
Middlesex HA1 3YJ
Helpline: 0845 608 4455 (Mon–Fri, 10am–4pm)
Tel (admin): 020 8423 9111 (Mon–Fri, 9am–5pm)
Fax: 020 8423 9119
Web site: www.patients-association.co.uk
Gives advice on patients' rights, complaints procedures and access to health services or appropriate self-help groups.

Prince's Foundation for Integrated Health
33–41 Dallington Road
London EC1V 0BB
Tel: 020 3119 3100
Fax: 020 3119 3101
Web site: www.fihealth.org.uk
Encourages conventional and complementary practitioners to work together to integrate their approaches to health care; provides information, education and research and development.

Psoriatic Arthropathy Alliance
PO Box 111
St Albans AL2 3JQ
Tel: 0870 770 3212
Fax: 0870 770 3213
Web site: www.paalliance.org
Raises awareness of psoriatic arthropathy. Provides information, produces a regular journal and puts people in touch with one another. You don't have to be a member if you wish to receive information.

RADAR (Royal Association for Disability and Rehabilitation)
12 City Forum
250 City Road
London EC1V 8AF
Tel: 020 7250 3222
Textphone: 020 7250 4119
Fax: 020 7250 0212
Web site: www.radar.org.uk
Information about aids and mobility, holidays, sport and leisure for disabled people. Campaigns to improve the rights and care of disabled people. Sells special key to access locked disabled toilets.

REMAP
National Organiser
'Hazeldene'
Ightham
Sevenoaks
Kent TN15 9AD
Tel: 0845 1300 456
Fax: 0845 1300 789
Web site: www.remap.org.uk
Makes or adapts aids, when not commercially available, for people with disabilities, at no charge to the disabled person. Has local branches.

St Thomas' Lupus Trust
The Rayne Institute
St Thomas' Hospital
London SE1 7EH
Tel: 020 7188 3562
Fax: 020 7188 3574
Web site: www.lupus.org.uk
Supports both research into lupus and the Louise Coote Lupus Unit and provides information both to professionals and to people who have the condition.

Glossary

Glossary

A

ACID REFLUX – Painful condition marked by stomach acid flowing back up into the oesophagus, leading to heartburn and gastrointestinal damage.

ACTIVE INGREDIENT – The element in a medication or supplement that performs the treatment function in the body, as opposed to inactive ingredients, which are fillers to give the product taste, shape or binding.

ACUTE – Lasting for a short or contained period of time, as opposed to pain or illness that is chronic, or long-lasting and possibly permanent.

ACUPUNCTURE – Medicine technique created in ancient China in which thin needles are used to puncture the body at specific sites along energy pathways call meridians. Widely considered a complementary therapy, but gaining acceptance in Western medicine for pain relief. *Acupressure* is another form of this treatment, but one involving hand pressure rather than needle punctures.

ADDICTION – Dangerous psycho-logical reliance on and use of a drug or other treatment.

ADRENALINE – Hormone produced by the adrenal glands near the kidneys. Adrenaline is produced during times of emotional or physical excitement.

ALEXANDER TECHNIQUE – Exercise-related movement therapy aimed at teaching the body less painful ways to move.

ALLOPATHIC – the term used for standard, orthodox medical treatment.

ANAEMIA – A condition of the blood in which red blood cells are in some way not operating to their required optimum level, perhaps due to a lack in their number or in their haemoglobin content.

ANAESTHESIA – A state induced by chemicals that induce a partial or complete loss of sensation and/or loss of consciousness. Used for temporary pain relief, or to reduce sensation for surgery and other medical procedures.

ANAESTHETIST – Doctor specializing in administering anaesthesia during surgical procedures or other medical treatment. This specialty includes the field of *pain medicine*, the comprehensive treatment of pain. Some anaesthetists are also pain medicine specialists.

ANALGESIC – A medication used to treat pain, including paracetamol and opiate drugs. *Topical analgesics*, or rub-on ointments that temporarily treat pain, are included in this category.

ANKYLOSING SPONDYLITIS (AS) – A form of arthritis that mainly affects the spine and sacroiliac joints (at the base of the spine where it attaches to the pelvis). In severe cases, people with AS may develop a fused and rigid spine.

ANTICONVULSANTS – Medicines designed to suppress convulsions.

ANTIBODIES – Cells that help the body's immune system fight against foreign agents that may cause disease.

ANTIPYRETIC – Medicines designed to lower raised body temperature, or fever.

ANTISPASMODICS – Medicines designed to suppress muscle spasms or seizures.

AROMATHERAPY – Complementary therapy involving the inhaling or application of particular scented substances (such as plant oils) in order to promote relaxation.

ARTHRODESIS – A surgical procedure in which the two bones that form a joint are prepared and held in place, allowing them to fuse into a single, immovable unit.

ARTHROPLASTY – Also called joint replacement surgery, a procedure in which a damaged joint is surgically removed and replaced with a synthetic one.

ARTHROSCOPY – Surgical procedure in which a thin, illuminated scope is inserted into the joint through a small incision, allowing the joint's interior to be viewed on a monitor or screen.

ARTHROSCOPE – Instrument used in arthroscopy to view the inside of the joint.

ASPIRATION – The process of removing fluid or cells from the body through a needle. Often used in removing fluid from joints in a variety of diagnostic tests and treatment procedures.

ATROPHY – A decrease in muscle mass, or wasting, due to extended lack of use or immobility.

AUTOANTIBODIES – Antibodies that attack the body's own cells instead of the foreign cells that may cause disease.

AUTOIMMUNE DISEASE – A disease in which the immune system, which is designed to protect the body from foreign invaders such as viruses and bacteria, instead turns against itself and

Glossary

causes damage to the body's healthy tissue.

AUTONOMIC NERVES – Nerves that regulate basic body functions, such as heart rate, breathing, sweating, blood pressure and bowel function.

AYURVEDA – Healing tradition created in ancient India and incorporating various healing philosophies and techniques, including yoga.

B

BALNEOTHERAPY – Therapeutic use of warm, mineral-rich mud through the application of packs or soaking in baths.

BENIGN – A term for a tumour or mass that is non-cancerous.

BIOFEEDBACK – The use of electronic instruments to measure body functions and feed that information back to you, allowing you to learn how to control body processes, such as heart rate or blood pressure, that are generally thought to be out of conscious control.

BIOLOGICAL RESPONSE MODIFIERS – Agents derived from living sources, as opposed to synthesized chemicals, that target specific immune-system chemicals that play a role in the inflammation and damage caused by a disease while leaving other immune-system components intact.

BIOPSY – A test performed on a piece of body tissue that is removed surgically, most often through a small incision. The tissue is then examined by a pathologist. Your doctor may use a biopsy to diagnose diseases of the joint, muscle, skin or blood vessels.

BISPHOSPHONATES – A class of medications that inhibit bone resorption and are used to treat bone diseases such as osteoporosis.

BONE RESORPTION – The loss of bone through physiological means. In the body, existing bone is constantly being resorbed while new bone grows to take its place. Bone resorption is essential to healthy bones, but it may outpace the growth of new bone.

BONE SPUR – A protruding outgrowth of bone, commonly on the heel, caused by disease or injury.

BRACE – A medical device used to hold a joint in place for proper movement, offering additional support for weak joints or muscles. Braces can be a temporary aid for reducing some pain.

BURSA – Small, fluid-filled sac that cushions and lubricates joints. Plural is bursae.

BURSITIS – Inflammation of a bursa.

C

CAPSAICIN – Substance derived from the oil of hot cayenne peppers and used as a topical analgesic.

CARPAL TUNNEL SYNDROME – Painful neuropathic condition caused by compression and irritation of the median nerve located in the wrist.

CARTILAGE – Smooth, rubbery tissue covering the ends of the bones at the joints, allowing the joint to move smoothly.

CELL OXIDATION – The natural process of cells breaking down over time due to oxidation, or exposure to oxygen.

CENTRAL NERVOUS SYSTEM – The part of the body's nervous system that includes the brain and spinal cord, but not including the *peripheral nervous system*, or the network of nerves that spread throughout the body.

CEREBRAL CORTEX – The outer layer of grey matter of the brain.

CHINESE MEDICINE – Traditional Chinese healing philosophy and practices, including acupuncture, herbal treatments and qi gong.

CHIROPRACTIC – Practice of healing based on spinal manipulation and the belief that illness stems from misalignment of the spine.

CHIROPRACTOR – A practitioner of chiropractic, who has four years of specialized training in chiropractic.

CHRONIC – Lasting for a long time, usually defined as three months or more. Chronic pain and chronic conditions may also be permanent.

COLLAGEN – a protein that is the primary component of cartilage and other connective tissue

COMPLEMENTARY THERAPY – A therapy that is used in conjunction with standard medical therapies, but not in place of them. Can include healthy habits such as exercise, diet or relaxation techniques.

COMPLEX REGIONAL PAIN SYNDROME – See *reflex sympathetic dystrophy.*

CORTICOSTEROIDS – A group of hormones, including cortisol, produced by the adrenal glands. They can be

Glossary

synthetically produced (that is, made in a laboratory) and have powerful anti-inflammatory effects. They are sometimes called just steroids.

COUNTERIRRITANTS – Topical analgesics that contain stimulating or cooling substances meant to provide a soothing counteraction to localized pain. Often contain oil of wintergreen, camphor, menthol or other substances that create a sensation of coolness.

COX-2 SPECIFIC INHIBITOR – A type of non-steroidal anti-inflammatory drug (NSAID) that is designed to be safer for the stomach than other NSAIDs. COX-2 inhibitors work by inhibiting hormone-like substances in the body that cause pain and inflammation without interfering with similar substances that protect the stomach lining.

CRANIAL MANIPULATION – Application of gentle pressure to the skull (cranium) in an attempt to relieve a range of medical conditions. Usually performed by an osteopath or a chiropractor.

CRANIOSACRAL THERAPY – Complementary therapy involving physical manipulation of the head, neck and spine. The philosophy behind craniosacral therapy is that pain results from an imbalance of fluids in these body parts.

CYTOKINES – Chemical messengers in the body that play a role in the immune response.

D

DEGENERATIVE – A gradually worsening deterioration in the structure of a body part.

DEPENDENCE – A physical and/or emotional reliance on a drug that may be, in some cases, unhealthy. Differs from addiction, which connotes dangerous use of and psychological need for a drug.

DERMATOMYOSITIS – See *polymyositis*.

DEXA – Short for dual-energy X-ray absorptiometry, a scan that measures bone density at the hip and spine to diagnose osteoporosis and evaluate bone density.

DISABILITY – A state of being unable to perform basic functions. Also a legal term describing long-term, complete incapacity to work.

DMARDS – Short for disease-modifying antirheumatic drugs, a class of medications that work to modify the course of rheumatoid arthritis and other forms of inflammatory arthritis, slowing or even stopping its progression.

DOSAGE – The amount of a drug's active ingredient that a person consumes in one measured allotment.

DURA MATER – The outer membrane covering the spinal cord. There is a risk of puncturing the dura mater in some pain injection procedures.

E

EFFICACY – Effectiveness of a procedure or treatment.

ELECTROACUPUNCTURE – Acupuncture employing electronic stimulation of the needles used in the procedure.

ENDORPHINS AND ENKEPHALINS – Naturally occurring molecules, produced by the brain, that bind to opiate receptors and act as neuro-transmitters.

EPICONDYLE – The area of the bone where the muscles are attached to the elbow.

EPIDURAL ANAESTHESIA – Anaesthetic injected directly into the spinal canal, between the spinal column and the outermost cover of the spinal cord. Epidural anaesthesia is used to numb the lower half of the body and is often used in knee surgery. Some chronic pain patients receive *epidural injections* as well.

EROSIONS – Areas where a structure is worn away. In the gastrointestinal system, refers to shallow, small ulcers that develop in the lining of the stomach or intestine, causing intense pain. Erosions can also occur in joints in osteoarthritis and other forms of arthritis.

ERYTHROCYTE SEDIMENTATION RATE (ESR) – A test measuring how fast red blood cells (erythrocytes) clump together and fall to the bottom of a test tube like sediment.

F

FASCIA – Fibrous tissues located beneath the skin. Fascia can become inflamed and painful. Some massage techniques involve manipulation of the fascia.

FATIGUE – A generalized, long-lasting feeling of tiredness or sleepiness that isn't relieved by sleep or rest.

FIBROMYALGIA – A syndrome characterized by widespread muscle

Glossary

pain, the presence of tender points (or points on the body that feel painful on pressure) and often debilitating fatigue and other symptoms.

FIELD BLOCK INJECTIONS – Another term for trigger point injections, or injections of corticosteroid directly into points of the body that may be triggers for painful reactions elsewhere in the body.

FLARE – An unusually severe episode of disease activity.

FREE RADICAL – A compound that is unstable and a possible contributor to cell degeneration. Free radicals are in the atmosphere as well as the body.

G

GATE CONTROL THEORY OF PAIN – A theory that describes how, before pain signals may go from the peripheral nervous system on to the central nervous system, they have to pass through pain gates. These 'gates' open or close depending on a number of factors (including instructions coming from the brain) and affect the degree to which pain messages can reach the brain.

GOLFER'S ELBOW – Similar to tennis elbow, but when the inside of the elbow is affected. The medical term is medial epicondylitis.

GOUT – a form of arthritis that occurs when uric acid builds up in the blood and deposits as crystals in the joints and other tissue. A joint affected by gout may be excruciatingly painful and shiny and purplish in appearance.

GUIDED IMAGERY – Technique involving concentrated focus on pleasant images as a distraction from pain.

H

HAEMATOMA – A localized swelling or sac that is filled with blood.

HEALTH-CARE PROFESSIONAL – Generally, any registered professional involved with a patient about health-care concerns.

HELLERWORK – Massage-based complementary practice incorporating methods to teach the person to move or hold their body in a less painful way.

HERBAL SUPPLEMENTS – Nutritional supplements that contain natural plant-derived substances and are meant to have therapeutic or health-promoting effects. Herbal supplement is a loosely applied term.

HYALURONIC ACID – a substance in the synovial fluid of the joints that gives the fluid its viscosity and shock-absorbing properties.

HYDROTHERAPY – The use of water in the treatment of the effects of disease.

I

IDIOPATHIC PAIN – Pain of unknown cause or origin.

IN VITRO – Literally 'in glass', or in a test tube. A term describing a test performed in a test tube in a laboratory setting as opposed to being conducted in a clinical trial or on live creatures.

IN VIVO – Literally 'in the living'. A term describing something being done to live creatures, often referring to drug or supplement tests conducted in clinical trials on humans or animals.

IMMUNE SYSTEM – The body's natural system of defence against invaders, such as viruses and bacteria, that it sees as harmful.

IMPLANTABLE DEVICES – Pain-relief devices that are surgically implanted inside a person's body. Some implantable devices are pumps that deliver steady doses of analgesic medicine, and others are electrical devices that deliver steady pulses of electrical stimulation.

INFECTIOUS ARTHRITIS – Form of arthritis that occurs when an infection settles in a joint or joints.

INFLAMMATION – An immune-system response to injury or infection that causes heat, redness and swelling in the affected area. In some forms of arthritis, joint and organ inflammation occurs as a result of a faulty immune response to the body's own tissues.

INTEGRATIVE MEDICINE – Practice of incorporating complementary or natural medical techniques and therapies into a medical or allopathic philosophy of medicine.

INTERLEUKIN – A protein produced by the body that contributes to the inflammation iprocess.

INTRACTABLE PAIN – Pain that cannot be effectively treated or that is not responding to any available pain treatment.

INTRAMUSCULAR INJECTION – Injection of a medicine or solution into muscle tissue.

INTRATHECAL – The space around the spinal cord within the spinal canal.

Glossary

INTRAVENOUS – Into a vein. Some medicines are injected or infused intravenously.

J

JOINT – The juncture of two or more bones, whereby the bones are able to move in relation to each other.

JOINT CAPSULE – The thin fibrous membranous structure that surrounds a joint.

JUVENILE IDIOPATHIC ARTHRITIS – A type of arthritis that occurs in children under age 16. There are three different forms of JIA, differentiated primarily by the number of joints they affect.

L

LIGAMENTS – Bands of tough connective tissue that attach bones to bones and help keep them together at a joint.

LIMBIC CENTRE – A part of the brain near the brainstem where pain signals may be processed.

LYME DISEASE – A form of infectious arthritis caused by the person acquiring the *Borrelia burgdorferi* bacterium, usually from the bite of an infected tick.

M

MALIGNANT – Term for a tumour or mass that is cancerous.

MANIPULATION THERAPY – Complementary therapy involving the physical manipulation of a part of the body, such as the spine, neck or cranium.

MEDICAL HISTORY – Record of a patient's personal health background, including diseases, injuries, surgical procedures, vaccinations, health habits or health problems the patient may have had, as well as family history of disease.

MEDITATION – Practice of using deep breathing and concentration exercises in order to promote relaxation.

MERIDIANS – In Chinese medicine, energy pathways throughout the body that an acupuncturist uses to stimulate healthy energy flow or to reduce pain.

MESMERISM – Original term for hypnosis.

METHOTREXATE – A disease-modifying antirheumatic drug, used for treating autoimmune diseases such as rheumatoid arthritis.

MOXIBUSTION – A form of acupuncture employing a smouldering cone of dried herb, such as mugwort.

MOTOR NERVES – Nerves that carry messages from the brain to the muscles, allowing you to move various body parts.

MRI – Short for magnetic resonance imaging, MRI is a procedure in which a very strong magnet is used to pass a force through the body to create a clear, detailed image of a cross-section of the body.

MUCUS – Thick, lubricating or coating fluid produced by the membranes that line certain organs of the body.

MUSCLE – Fibrous tissue in the body holds us upright and gives the body movement, including both movement

that we consciously initiate (e.g. waving a hand) and movement of which we are scarcely aware (e.g. movement of the blood through the vessels or food through the digestive system).

N

NATURAL MEDICINE – Complementary field of health care involving treating illness or pain through herbs, supplements and various non-medical methods.

NERVE BLOCK INJECTIONS – Injection treatments involving the numbing of nerve fibres that may be the source of pain.

NERVE ENDINGS – Tiny structures at the end of nerves that sense pain, temperature, vibration or other stimuli. Includes the *nociceptors*, which perceive pain and other stimuli that might indicate harm to the body.

NERVOUS SYSTEM – The body's system of cells, tissues and organs that collect and distribute data using a complex series of chemical and electrical signals; includes nerves, the spinal cord and the brain.

NEUROLOGIST – Doctor specializing in diseases or problems of the nervous system.

NEUROPATHIC PAIN – Pain arising from within the nervous system.

NEUROPLASTICITY – The brain's ability to recover structurally and/or functionally after injury or disease.

NEUROSTIMULATORS – Devices surgically implanted in the body to deliver electrical signals that treat nerve-related pain.

Glossary

NEUROSURGEON – Doctor with specialized training in surgical treatment of the nervous system.

NEUROTRANSMITTER – A naturally occurring chemical in the nervous system, which transmits signals from one nerve cell to another.

NOCICEPTORS – Peripheral nerve endings that sense pain.

NON-STEROIDAL ANTI-INFLAMMATORY DRUGS (NSAIDS) – A class of medications commonly used to ease the pain and inflammation of many forms of arthritis.

NURSE – Health-care professional who assists doctors in many procedures, as well as administering many basic health-care treatments on his or her own.

NURSE PRACTITIONER – A registered nurse with additional training in a medical specialty.

O

OBESE – A term describing a person who is more than 20 per cent over their ideal body weight.

OCCUPATIONAL THERAPIST (OT) – A registered health-care professional who is trained to evaluate the impact of disease or injury on daily activities, and advise patients on easier ways to perform activities that put strain on damaged joints. May also prescribe splints and assistive devices.

OCCUPATIONAL THERAPY – Health-care field focusing on the patient's ability to perform tasks that may be impaired due to disease, surgery or injury, and training patients to find practical ways to do such tasks.

OPIATE – A drug derived from opium or opium-like substances that is used as a powerful analgesic, or pain reliever.

ORTHOPAEDIC SURGEON – A doctor specializing in surgery involving the musculoskeletal system, including bones and joints.

OSTEOARTHRITIS (OA) – The most common form of arthritis. OA causes cartilage breakdown at certain joints (including the spine, hands, hips and knees) resulting in pain and deformity.

OSTEOPATH – A registered practitioner who treats problems in the structure of the body using soft-tissue work and manipulation (osteopathy) to optimize the working of the internal organs.

OSTEOPOROSIS – A condition in which the body loses bone mass such that bones are susceptible to disabling fractures.

OSTEOTOMY – A surgical procedure that involves cutting and repositioning a bone, usually performed in cases of severe joint malalignment.

OVER THE COUNTER – A term describing drugs or treatments sold without a doctor's prescription.

P

PAIN CLINIC – Usually a large medical institution providing comprehensive treatment programmes for people in severe or chronic pain.

PAIN-MANAGEMENT PLAN – A comprehensive plan of treatments and strategies designed to help a person manage chronic pain.

PAIN MEDICINE – A subspecialty of anaesthesiology that focuses on treatment of pain, including chronic and severe acute pain.

PAIN REHABILITATION – The process of treating a person with chronic pain and assisting them in developing a long-term plan for managing life with chronic pain.

PARACETAMOL – The most commonly used analgesic medicine.

PERIPHERAL NERVOUS SYSTEM – The network of nerves throughout the body that connects the central nervous system (the brain and spinal cord) to organs, blood vessels, muscles, glands and other parts of the body.

PHYSIOTHERAPIST (PHYSIO) – A health-care professional who uses physical approaches to promote, maintain and restore physical and social well-being.

PHYSIOTHERAPY – Health-care field focusing on exercise and rehabilitation to reduce pain and restore movement following disease, surgery or injury.

PILATES – Exercise technique involving specific postures and stretches designed to strengthen the core muscles.

PLACEBO EFFECT – The phenomenon in which a person receiving an inactive drug or therapy experiences a reduction in symptoms because he or she believes it to be a genuine treatment.

PLANTAR FASCIITIS – A painful condition in which the thick, fibrous tissue stretching across the sole of your foot, from the heel to the toes, becomes inflamed.

Glossary

POLYMYALGIA RHEUMATICA – a disease causing joint and muscle pain in the neck, shoulders and hips and a general feeling of malaise. The disease is usually marked by a high ESR (see *erythrocyte sedimentation rate*) and occasionally by a fever.

POLYMYOSITIS – An arthritis-related disease in which generalized weakness results from inflammation of the muscles, primarily those of the shoulders, upper arms, thighs and hips. When a skin rash accompanies muscle weakness, the disease is called dermatomyositis.

PRACTICE NURSE AND NURSE PRACTITIONER – Practice nurses and nurse practitioners are registered nurses with advanced training and emphasis in primary care, who can diagnose illness and, in some cases, prescribe medication.

PRACTITIONER – A person who performs various complementary therapies as a vocation or profession.

PRIMARY-CARE DOCTOR – Doctor who provides general health care to a patient. Also known as a general practitioner (GP).

PROLOTHERAPY – Surgical therapy involving the injection of a chemical irritant into painful soft tissues in order to stimulate blood flow into the affected area and promote healing.

PROSTAGLANDINS – Hormone-like substances in the body that play a role in pain and inflammation, among other body functions.

PSORIATIC ARTHRITIS – A form of arthritis that is accompanied by the skin disease psoriasis.

PURINE – One of the two classes of bases involved in the makeup of DNA and RNA; an end-product of purine processing is uric acid. Eating foods rich in purines may contribute to the development of gout; these foods include organ meats, game and shellfish.

Q

QI GONG – An Asian practice that incorporates meditation, breathing exercises and movement to promote health and self-healing.

R

RADIOGRAPH – Another name for X-ray.

RADIOLOGIST – A doctor who specializes in conducting and examining imaging tests for diagnosis.

RANGE OF MOTION – The distance and angles at which your joints can be moved, extended and rotated in various directions.

RAYNAUD'S PHENOMENON – A condition in which the blood vessels in the hands go into spasm in response to stress or cold temperatures, resulting in pain, tingling, numbness and colour change.

RECEPTORS – The parts of sensory nerves that receive and respond to various stimuli.

REFLEX SYMPATHETIC DYSTROPHY – A chronic pain condition marked by burning pain, swelling and tenderness of an extremity, rising from irritation or damage to nerves in that area. Also known as complex regional pain syndrome.

REFLEXOLOGY – Complementary therapy based on a philosophy that applying pressure to particular points on the feet can have a beneficial effect on other, distant parts of the body.

REM SLEEP – Stage of sleep marked by 'rapid eye movement' in which a person dreams.

RESECTION – A surgical procedure that involves removing all or part of a bone, sometimes used to relieve joint pain and stiffness.

REYE'S SYNDROME – Dangerous, possibly fatal acute condition associated with the use of aspirin in certain situations, particularly in children. People developing Reye's syndrome may develop swelling of the brain and enlargement of the liver.

RHEUMATIC DISEASE – A general term referring to conditions characterized by pain and stiffness of the joints or muscles. There are more than 200 rheumatic diseases. The term is often used interchangeably with 'arthritis' (meaning joint inflammation), but not all rheumatic diseases affect the joints or involve inflammation.

RHEUMATISM – A term used loosely (though not as widely used as it was in the past) to refer to conditions that cause pain and swelling in the joints and supporting tissues.

RHEUMATOID ARTHRITIS – A chronic inflammatory form of arthritis in which the body's otherwise protective immune system turns against the body and attacks tissues of the joints, causing pain, inflammation and deformity.

RHEUMATOID FACTOR (RF) – A blood protein (antibody) that is found in high

Glossary

levels in many people with rheumatoid arthritis. It is often associated with RA severity or disease activity, and its presence can be helpful to a doctor in making a diagnosis.

1 – A doctor who specializes in treating arthritis and related diseases, also known as rheumatic diseases. A *paediatric rheumatologist* specializes in treating rheumatic diseases in children.

ROTATOR CUFF – A grouping of four tendons that attach to and stabilize the shoulder joints; these tendons can become inflamed and painful through injury or overuse.

S

SACROILIAC JOINTS – The joints where the spine attaches to the pelvis.

SALICYLATES – A subcategory of non-steroidal anti-inflammatory drugs (NSAIDs), which includes aspirin. Also describes topical creams containing salicylic acid that relieve pain and inflammation.

SCIATICA – Painful condition involving inflammation of or pressure on the sciatic nerve, one of the body's largest nerves, which runs from the lower back through the buttocks, with branches extending down the back of the legs to the feet. Sciatica pain is often felt in the buttock and at the back of the thigh.

SCLERODERMA – An umbrella term for several diseases that involve the abnormal growth of connective tissue. In most cases, the effects of this overgrowth are limited to the skin and underlying tissues, but in others, tissue overgrowth can affect the joints, blood vessels and internal organs.

SELF-MANAGEMENT – The process of a person taking an active role in managing his or her own pain or disease, through self-monitoring of health, lifestyle modification, diet, exercise and other means.

SENSORY NERVES – Nerves that convert stimuli (e.g. pressure, temperature and vibration) from the environment into electrical impulses that they convey to the spinal cord.

SHIATSU – Japanese massage technique that is similar to acupressure, but also incorporating stretching techniques.

SHOCK-WAVE THERAPY – Complementary therapy involving use of ultrasound technology.

SOFT-TISSUE RHEUMATIC SYNDROMES – Painful conditions affecting the soft tissues of the body.

SONOGRAMS – Images created through ultrasonography.

SPECIALIST – A doctor with additional years of training in a specialized field of medicine. Specialists include ortho-paedic surgeons, rheumatologists, cardiologists, anaesthetists, etc.

SPINAL CORD – Thick cord of nerve tissue that runs from the base of the brain down the spinal canal.

SPINAL CORD STIMULATION – Electronic stimulation of the spinal cord through an implanted electronic device as a way to relieve pain.

SPINAL MANIPULATION – Physical adjustment of the vertebrae of the spine, particularly in chiropractic or osteopathic treatment.

SPLINT – Device used to support or stabilize a joint or to position a joint in a way that prevents further pain or injury to the joint or the soft tissues surrounding it.

STEROIDS – See *corticosteroids*.

SUBCUTANEOUS – Just beneath the skin. Some medicines are injected subcutaneously, beneath the skin.

SUBDERMAL – Beneath the dermal layer of the skin; a deeper level than subcutaneous.

SUBSTANCE P – A substance present in the brain, believed to be a transmitter of pain impulses.

SYMPTOM – Any sensation or change in bodily function that is experienced by the patient and is associated with a particular disease.

SYNAPSE – Gap between nerve cells.

SYNOVECTOMY – Surgical removal of a diseased joint lining (see also *synovium*).

SYNOVIAL FLUID – A slippery liquid secreted by the synovium that lubricates the joint, making movement easier.

SYNOVIUM – A thin membrane that lines the joint capsule and can become inflamed in rheumatoid arthritis.

SYNTHETIC – Manmade or made in a laboratory, as opposed to naturally occurring.

SYSTEMIC – A term used to refer to anything that affects the whole body.

Glossary

T

T'AI CHI – An ancient Chinese practice that involves gentle, fluid movements and meditation to help strengthen muscles, improve balance and relieve stress.

TARSAL TUNNEL SYNDROME – Similar to carpal tunnel syndrome, only involving a nerve in the instep of the foot.

TENDER POINTS – Specific, precise areas on the body that are particularly painful upon the application of slight pressure. The finding of tender points is useful in the diagnosis of fibromyalgia.

TENDER POINT EXAMINATION – Examination of the patient's tender points to determine a diagnosis of fibromyalgia.

TENDINITIS – Inflammation of the tendons.

TENDONS – Thick connective tissues that attach the muscles to the bones.

TENNIS ELBOW – A common term for lateral epicondylitis, an inflammation of the epicondyle – the area of the bone where the muscles are attached to the elbow.

TENS – Transcutaneous electrical nerve stimulation, a treatment for pain that uses a small device to direct mild electric pulses to nerves in a painful area.

THALAMUS – The part of the brain where pain messages are first processed.

THERAPEUTIC DRUGS – Medications used to treat illness or pain.

TINNITUS – Chronic ringing in the ears. Causes vary, including adverse reactions to drugs, injury or infection.

TOLERANCE – A gradually developed resistance to the effectiveness of a drug, leading to the need for higher doses of the drug for continued effectiveness.

TOPHI – Nodes or masses of crystallized uric acid that settle in various joints in people with gout.

TRANSDERMAL PATCH – Small, self-adhering square of plastic that delivers sustained dose of medication that is absorbed through the skin.

TRIGGER FINGER – Stenosing tenosynovitis, a condition involving a thickening of the lining around the tendons in the fingers, causing the finger to lock in a painful, bent position and then to snap open suddenly.

TUINA – Chinese massage technique involving manipulation of pressure points.

TUMOUR – A mass of tissue growth in the body that is distinct from its surrounding structures. May be benign (harmless) or malignant (cancerous).

TUMOUR NECROSIS FACTOR (TNF) – A cytokine (chemical messenger) in the body that plays a role in inflammation and tissue destruction in diseases such as rheumatoid arthritis, but is also important for normal function of the immune system. Blocking TNF with biological response modifiers has proven to ease symptoms and inhibit joint destruction in RA.

U

URIC ACID – A bodily waste product that is excreted through the kidneys. When the body produces too much uric acid or doesn't excrete it efficiently, excess uric acid can deposit as crystals in the joint and other tissues, a condition known as gout (see Gout).

URINALYSIS – The analysis of urine using physical, chemical and microscopic tests to detect the presence of infection, levels of uric acid excreted or abnormal constituents.

V

VASCULITIS – Inflammation of the blood vessels that can be a complication of some forms of inflammatory forms of arthritis and related conditions.

VISCOSUPPLEMENTS – Products injected into osteoarthritic joints (particularly the knee) to replace hyaluronic acid that usually gives the joint fluid its viscosity. Also known as joint fluid therapy.

W

WHIPLASH – Painful condition resulting from the neck being whipped back and forth sharply, usually during a fall or motor vehicle accident.

Y

YOGA – An ancient Indian practice that involves a series of body postures and includes exercise, meditation and breathing components to improve posture and balance and help relieve stress on the joints, as well as emotional stress.

Index

Index

Page numbers in *italic* indicate an
illustration or table; numbers followed
by *g* indicate an entry in the Glossary

Index

death (avascular necrosis) 83
density scans 38
fusion 101–2
nociceptors in 9–10
resection 102, 204*g*
resorption 199*g*
scans 40–1
spurs 15, 38, 199*g*
thinning *see* osteoporosis
borage 124, 134
Borrelia burgdorferi test 37
Boswellia serrata (frankincense) 121
Botox (botulinum toxin) injections 99
brace 44, 199*g*
brain
   dealing with pain 21
   recognizing pain 10, 147–8
   stimulation, deep 102
brand names for drugs 57
breathing, deep 181
bromelain 121
Brufen 75, 76
buprenorphine 73, 74
burns from heat or cold treatment 159
bursae 15, 199*g*
   inflammation 16
   injections into 99
bursitis 16, 76, 199*g*
   treatment 84

C

C-reactive protein test 36
calcification, diagnosis 38
calcium deposits in bursae 16
calcium supplements 126, 134, 135
camphor 73
cancer cells 86
Cannabis sativa 153
caplet 60
capsaicin 73, 199*g*
capsule 60
carbamazepine 69, 92
Carisoma 92
carisoprodol 92
carpal tunnel syndrome 16–17, 76, 199*g*
   treatment 84
carrying loads 161
cartilage 199*g*
   breaking down 15, 97, 120
   shark 126
CAT (CT) scans 39–40

cataracts from corticosteroids 85
catheter 107
cat's claw 121
Celebrex 79
celecoxib 79
cell
   abnormally dividing 86
   oxidation 134, 199*g*
central nervous system 9, 199*g*
central pain syndrome, treatment 92, 103
cerebral cortex 12, 199*g*
cetyl myristoleate (CMO) 122
chickenpox, risks of 85
Childers, Norman F 133–4
children
   aspirin and 67
   pain and 19
   rheumatologist for 26
Chinese medicine 140, 199*g*
chiropodist 28
chiropractic 44, 142, 199*g*
chiropractor 28, 199*g*
choline salicylate 76
chondroitin 97–8, 120–1
   shark cartilage 126
   side effects 121
chronic pain 2, 3
   causes 11
   definition 199*g*
   opiates 73
   perception 20
   treatment 24
   types 8, 18
ciclosporin 87
cimetidine 77
Cipramil 91
citalopram 91
Clinoril 76
clonaxepam 69
CMO (cetyl myristoleate) 122
co-codamol 72
codeine 69, 72
colchicine 89
cold treatment 69, 158–60
collagen 120, 199*g*
   supplements 122, 126
communication with doctor 8, 20, 25, 32
   about complementary therapy 116
   about drugs 57, 63, 78
complement test 36

complementary therapy 44, 140–54, 199*g*
   controversies 114
   definition 112–13
   doing your own research 115–16
   efficacy tests 118
   evaluation 115–17
   herbs and supplements 112–36
   practitioners 140
   regulation and development 114
   research studies 118–19
   risks 113–14, 117–18
complex regional pain syndrome *see* reflex sympathetic dystrophy
compression treatment 69
computed axial tomography (CT scans) 39–40
Corrisone 83
connective tissues, prolotherapy for 150–1
corticosteroids 24, 82–5, 199–200*g*
   dosages 84, 85
   injections 98–9
   methods of taking 84–5
   side effects 83, 85, 98
   steroid treatment card 83
   surgery and 103
cortisol 82, 83, 179
cortisone 85
Cortone Acetate 85
counterirritants 73, 200*g*
COX-1 76, 77
COX-2 specific inhibitors 76, 77–9, 200*g*
   side effects 78
cranial manipulation 144, 200*g*
cranial rhizotomy 102
craniosacral therapy 144, 200*g*
Cremalgin 74
Crohn's disease, treatment 82, 86
CT scans 39–40
Cuprofen 74
cyclooxygenase *see* COX
cysts, diagnosing 41–2
cytokines 200*g*
   blocking 87
Cytotec 77

D

dairy foods 132
dancing 170–2
de Quervain's tendinitis 16

Index

Index

Index

Index

Index

Index

salsalate 76
salt 133
SAM-e 125
Sandimmun 87
sciatica 18, 205*g*
   epidural injections 100
   prolotherapy 150
scleroderma 205*g*
   diagnosis 36
scurvy 135
sea algae 125–6
seasonings 133
selective serotonin uptake inhibitors
      (SSRIs) 91
selenium 135
self-help for pain relief 158–74
self-management 2, 3–4, 205*g*
self-massage 160
sensitization to pain 11
sensory cortex 10, 12
sensory nerves 205*g*
serotonin 11
   abnormal production 90
Seroxat 91
sertraline 91
shark cartilage 126
shiatsu massage 145, 205*g*
shingles
   risks of 85
   treatment for pain 92
shock-wave therapy 150, 205*g*
shoulder
   circle exercise *165*
   rotator cuff tendinitis 16
side bend exercise in water 172
side effects 21, 62
   anticonvulsants 92–3
   biological response modifiers 88
   chondroitin and glucosamine 121
   corticosteroids 83, 85, 98
   COX-2 specific inhibitors 77–9
   DMARDs 86–7
   gout drugs 89
   implantable devices 108–9
   injection therapy 97
   mexiletine 93
   muscle relaxants 92
   NSAIDs 75, 76–7
   opiates 72
   topical analgesics 73–4
   tricyclic antidepressants 91
Sinequan 91

Sjögren's syndrome 18, 28
skeletal muscle relaxants 91–*2*
skin
   irritation from oils 152
   nerves in 9–10
skinrolling technique 146
SLE *see* lupus
sleep
   regulation of cycle 129
   REM 90, 204*g*
   therapy 129–30
sodium aurothiomalate 87
sodium salicylate 76
sodium valproate 69
soft tissue
   masses, diagnosis 38
   rheumatic syndromes 16, 76, 205*g*
   treatment 84–5
   scanning 38–9
Solonaceae vegetables 132–3
Solu-Cortef 85
somatic pain 13
somatic system 9
sonograms 205*g*
specialist 205*g*
spinal cord 205*g*
   electrodes 108
   intrathecal drug delivery pumps 108
   pain signals to 10
   stimulation 108–9, 205*g*
spinal dorsal rhizotomy 102
spinal manipulation 142, 143, 205*g*
spinal nerve blocks 99–100
spine, ankylosing spondylitis 18
splints 44, 205*g*
spray and stretch technique 146
sprays 61
SSRIs (selective serotonin uptake
      inhibitors), for fibromyalgia 91
St John's wort 129
stenosing tenosynovitis *see* trigger
      finger
steroids *see* corticosteroids
Still, Andrew 143
stinging nettle 126
strength and fitness, surgery and 103–4
stress 44–5
   causes 178–9, 180
   coping strategies 180
   definition 178
   reduction 178–85
   relaxation techniques 179–85

   responding to 180
   signs 179
stress journal 180–1, 184–5
stroke from COX-2 drugs 79
subcutaneous, definition 205*g*
subdermal, definition 205*g*
substance P 10, 12, 90, 205*g*
sulfasalazine 87
sulfinpyrazole 89
sulindac 76
   supplements *see* herbs and
      supplements
support stockings 104
suppository 61
surgery
   for diagnostic purposes 41–2
   for pain relief 100–5
      deciding on 103–6
   medications following 103, 105
suspensions 61
Swedish massage 145
sympathectomy 102
sympathetic pain 13
sympathetic spinal nerve block
      injections 100
symptoms, definition 205*g*
synapse 11, 205*g*
Synflex 75, 76
synovectomy 102, 205*g*
synovial fluid 15, 97, 205*g*
synovitis 75
synovium 15, 205*g*
synthetic, definition 205*g*
Synvec 98
systemic, definition 205*g*
systemic lupus erythematosus (SLE)
      see lupus

T

Tagamet 77
t'ai chi 173, 206*g*
Tanacetum parthenium (feverfew) 123
tarsal tunnel syndrome 17, 206*g*
Teejel 76
Tegretol 92
temporomandibular joint disorder 28
tender points 16, 35, 206*g*
   examination 34–5, 206*g*
   treatment 85
tendinitis 16, 76, 206*g*
   treatment 84

Index

tendons 15, 206*g*
tennis elbow 17, 76, 206*g*
TENS 69, 147, 206*g*
tension 44–5
tests for diagnosis 32
thalamus 10, 12, 102, 206*g*
therapeutic drugs 206*g*
thermal wraps 159
thermography 40–1
thumb, inflammation 16
thunder god vine 126
Tiger Balm 74
tinnitus 144, 206*g*
tissue typing test 37
TNF *see* tumour necrosis factor
tolerance, definition 206*g*
tomatoes 132
tophi 89, 206*g*
topical agents 61
    analgesics 73–4
toxins 133
traditional medicine *see*
      complementary therapy
tramadol 72, 91
transcutaneous electrical nerve
    stimulation *see* TENS
transdermal patch 75, 206*g*
treatment *see under* pain *(general only)*
triamcinolone 84, 85
tricyclic antidepressants
    for fibromyalgia 91
    side effects 91
    taken with muscle relaxants 92
trigeminal rhizotomy 102
trigger finger 17, 206*g*
    treatment 85
trigger point
    injections 99
    massage 145
Tripterygium wilfordii Hook F (thunder
    god vine) 126

tuina 145, 206*g*
tumour 206*g*
    diagnosis 38, 41–2
tumour necrosis factor (TNF) 206*g*
    blocking 87
turmeric 127

U

ulcers from NSAIDs 76
ultrasonography 41
ultrasound therapy 150
Uncaria tomentosa (cat's claw) 121
uric acid 206*g*
    accumulation causing gout 17, 89
    lowering levels 130
    testing for 36–7, 37
urinalysis 37, 206*g*

V

valerian root 129
vasculitis 206*g*
    diagnosis 36
vegetarian diet 133
vibrating balls 160
Vioxx 79
visceral pain 13
viscosupplements 97, 206*g*
visualization 148, 183
vitamins 130, 134–6
    vitamin A 135
    vitamin B 135
    vitamin C 135
    vitamin D 135
    vitamin E 135
    vitamin K 135
Voltarol 74, 76

W

walking 169–70, 171
warfarin, herbal products and 112
water exercise 149, 170
water jets 159
weight problems 32
    arthritis and 131
    controlling 162–3
    gout and 131
    surgery and 103
weight training 169
whiplash 150, 206*g*
white blood cells, levels 36
WHO 3-step analgesic ladder 67
willow bark 127
wintergreen 73
wood spider 122–3
wrist
    bending exercise *166*
    injections 84
    median nerve inflammation 16–17

X

X-rays 37–8
    risks 39

Y

yoga 173, 206*g*

Z

Zantac 77
zinc supplements 134
Zoton 77
Zyloric 89